Shoulder Concepts 2013: Consensus and Concerns

Guillermo Arce · Klaus Bak
Kevin P. Shea · Felix Savoie III
William Benjamin Kibler
Eiji Itoi · Augustus D. Mazzocca
Knut Beitzel · Emilio Calvo
Benno Ejnisman
Editors

Shoulder Concepts 2013: Consensus and Concerns

Proceedings of the ISAKOS Upper Extremity Committees 2009–2013

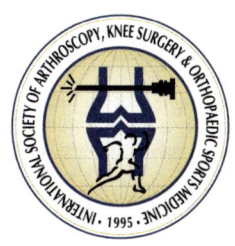

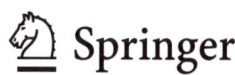

Editors

Guillermo Arce
Department of Orthopaedic Surgery
Instituto Argentino de Diagnóstico y Tratamiento
Buenos Aires
Argentina

Klaus Bak
Parkens Private Hospital
Copenhagen
Denmark

Kevin P. Shea
Health Center
University of Connecticut
Farmington, CT
USA

Felix Savoie III
School of Medicine
Tulane University
New Orleans, LA
USA

William Benjamin Kibler
Shoulder Center of Kentucky
Lexington, KY
USA

Eiji Itoi
Department of Orthopaedic Surgery
Tohoku University School of Medicine
Sendai, Miyagi
Japan

Augustus D. Mazzocca
Knut Beitzel
Department of Orthopaedic Surgery
Health Center
University of Connecticut
Farmington, CT
USA

Emilio Calvo
Shoulder and Elbow Reconstructive Surgery Unit
Department of Orthopedic Surgery
Fundacion Jimenez Diaz
Madrid
Spain

Benno Ejnisman
CETE-UNIFESP-EPM
São Paulo, SP
Brazil

ISBN 978-3-642-38096-9   ISBN 978-3-642-38097-6 (eBook)
DOI 10.1007/978-3-642-38097-6
Springer Heidelberg New York Dordrecht London

Library of Congress Control Number: 2013937196

© ISAKOS 2013
This work is subject to copyright. All rights are reserved by the Publisher, whether the whole or part of the material is concerned, specifically the rights of translation, reprinting, reuse of illustrations, recitation, broadcasting, reproduction on microfilms or in any other physical way, and transmission of information storage and retrieval, electronic adaptation, computer software, or by similar or dissimilar methodology now known or hereafter developed. Exempted from this legal reservation are brief excerpts in connection with reviews or scholarly analysis or material supplied specifically for the purpose of being entered and executed on a computer system, for exclusive use by the purchaser of the work. Duplication of this publication or parts thereof is permitted only under the provisions of the Copyright Law of the Publisher's location, in its current version, and permission for use must always be obtained from Springer. Permissions for use may be obtained through RightsLink at the Copyright Clearance Center. Violations are liable to prosecution under the respective Copyright Law.
The use of general descriptive names, registered names, trademarks, service marks, etc. in this publication does not imply, even in the absence of a specific statement, that such names are exempt from the relevant protective laws and regulations and therefore free for general use.
While the advice and information in this book are believed to be true and accurate at the date of publication, neither the authors nor the editors nor the publisher can accept any legal responsibility for any errors or omissions that may be made. The publisher makes no warranty, express or implied, with respect to the material contained herein.

Printed on acid-free paper

Springer is part of Springer Science+Business Media (www.springer.com)

Preface

On behalf of the International Society of Arthroscopy, Knee Surgery, and Orthopedic Sports Medicine (ISAKOS), we are proud to introduce a new edition of ISAKOS topical booklets. This booklet called '*Shoulder Concepts 2013: Consensus and Concerns*', represents an international cooperation of experts surgeons and lead researchers in the field. This issue provides a state-of-the-art review on several shoulder key topics such as a thorough assessment of the shoulder classifications along with the management of acromio-clavicular joint disorders and rotator cuff disease. Fortunately, ISAKOS partnership with Springer publishing continues to grow and produce relevant topical booklets, and we are honored that we were given the opportunity to participate. Certainly, the present booklet will prove very resourceful to orthopedic surgeons treating patients with shoulder disorders. We are deeply indebted to ISAKOS, Springer, and the authors for the extraordinary commitment to achieve this fruitful publication. We look forward to many more successful topical booklets in the future.

Guillermo Arce
Klaus Bak
Knut Beitzel
Kevin Shea
Eiji Itoi
Felix Savoie
William Benjamin Kibler
Augustus Mazzocca
Emilio Calvo
Benno Ejnisman

Contents

Part I ISAKOS Shoulder Terminology Project; Preliminary Report; Classifications and Scoring Systems

1 **Introduction**... 3
Kevin P. Shea and Guillermo Arce

2 **A Review of Rotator Cuff Classifications in Current Use**....... 5
Paulo Santoro Belangero, Benno Ejnisman and Guillermo Arce

3 **ISAKOS Classification System for Rotator Cuff Tears**.......... 15
Emilio Calvo and the ISAKOS Upper Extremity
and Anthroscopy Committees

4 **Review of Current Classifications of Shoulder Instability**....... 25
Kevin P. Shea

5 **ISAKOS Consensus Shoulder Instability Classification System**... 29
Kevin P. Shea

6 **Outcomes Scores for Shoulder Instability and Rotator
Cuff Disease**.. 35
Guillermo Arce and Kevin P. Shea

Part II Copenhagen Consensus on Acromio-Clavicular Disorders

7 **Copenhagen Consensus on Acromio-Clavicular Disorders**...... 51
Klaus Bak, Augustus Mazzocca, Knut Beitzel, Eiji Itoi,
Emilio Calvo, Guillermo Arce, William B. Kibler
and Raffy Mirzayan and the ISAKOS Upper Extremity Committee

**Part III Buenos Aires Consensus on Rotator Cuff Disease:
Known Facts and Unresolved Issues**

8   **Anatomy (Bone, Tendon, Bursa and Neurovascular Anatomy)** ...   71
    Felix Savoie, Eiji Itoi and Guillermo Arce

9   **Biomechanics**   77
    Ben Kibler and Giovanni Di Giacomo

10 **Tendinosis, Impingement and Ruptures**   81
    Klaus Bak, Eiji Itoi, Augustus Mazzocca and Tom Ludvigsen

11 **Arthroscopy and Repair**   87
    Jaap Willems, Dan Guttmann, Guillermo Arce and Greg Bain

12 **Augments and Prosthesis**   95
    Felix Savoie III, John Uribe, Matthew Provencher,
    Francisco Vergara and Emilio Calvo

Members of the ISAKOS Upper Extremity Committee

Guillermo R. Arce, Instituto Argentino de Diagnóstico y Tratamiento, Buenos Aires, Argentina, e-mail: guillermorarce@ciudad.com.ar

Gregory Ian Bain, University of Adelaide, North Adelaide, Australia, e-mail: greg@gregbain.com.au

Klaus Bak, Copenhagen Oe, Denmark, e-mail: kb@ppho.dk

Emilio Calvo, Shoulder and Elbow Reconstructive Surgery Unit, Madrid, Spain, e-mail: ECALVO@FJD.ES

Giovanni Di Giacomo, Concordia Hospital for Special Surgery, Rome, Italy, e-mail: concordia@iol.it

Benno Ejnisman, CETE-UNIFESP-EPM, São Paulo, Brazil, e-mail: bennoale@uol.com.br

Vicente Gutierrez, Clinica Las Condes, Santiago, Chile, e-mail: pacatoto@manquehue.net

Dan Guttmann, Taos Orthopaedic Institute, Taos, USA, e-mail: drg@taosortho.com

Eiji Itoi, Sendai, Japan, e-mail: itoi-eiji@med.tohoku.ac.jp

William Benjamin Kibler, Shoulder Center of Kentucky, Lexington, USA, e-mail: wkibler@aol.com

Tom Clement Ludvigsen, Oslo University Hospital, Oslo, Norway, e-mail: tomcl@ getmail.no

Augustus D. Mazzocca, University Of Connecticut Health Center, Farmington, USA, e-mail: mazzocca@uchc.edu

Alberto Castro Pochini, UNIFESP—Universidade Federal de Sao Paulo, Sao Paulo, Brazil, e-mail: apochini@uol.com.br

Matthew T. Provencher, Naval Medical Center San Diego, Coronado, USA, e-mail: mattprovencher@earthlink.net

Felix Henry Savoie III, Tulane University School of Medicine, New Orleans, USA, e-mail: fsavoie@tulane.edu

Hiroyuki Sugaya, Funabashi Orthopaedic Sports Medicine Center, Funabashi, Japan, e-mail: hsugaya@nifty.com

John William Uribe, UHZ Sports Medicine Institute, Coral Gables, USA, e-mail: johnu@baptisthealth.net

Francisco Javier Vergara, MEDS Sport Medicine Center, Santiago, Chile, e-mail: franciscoverg@gmail.com

W. Jaap Willems, Bergen, Netherland, e-mail: w.j.willems@xs4all.nl

Yon-Sik Yoo, Hallym University Hospital, Seoul, Korea, e-mail: yooo@hallym.ac.kr

Part I
ISAKOS Shoulder Terminology Project; Preliminary Report; Classifications and Scoring Systems

Introduction

Kevin P. Shea and Guillermo Arce

Rotator cuff disorders and shoulder instability are the most common causes of shoulder pain in our patient population. The incidence of first-time anterior shoulder dislocation is estimated to be between 8 and 24 per 100,000 person-years. Approximately, 300,000 to 400,000 rotator cuff surgeries are performed each year in the United States. Understanding the classification of the different types of injuries and the treatments that lead to the best outcomes for each is very important to the treating surgeon.

Most surgeons rely on their training and understanding of the published literature in recommending treatment for their patients with these shoulder disorders. Unfortunately, the literature contains studies that often give results that are contradictory, creating confusion about the best treatment recommendations. There are many reason cited for these differing recommendations. Many studies are retrospective and subject to missing data or high drop-out rates. Some contain only a small number of patients, and are under powered, possibly resulting in flawed conclusions. Meta-analysis methodology and critical reviews have attempted to better analyze the literature by combining similar studies in order to include more patients. However, these individual studies often use different classification systems and outcome assessments and are not directly comparable.

A better understanding of optimal treatment methods could be achieved by surgeons from different centers throughout the world pooling their data to achieve

K. P. Shea
University of Connecticut Health Center, Farmington Avenue 263, Farmington, CT 06034-4037, USA
e-mail: shea@uchc.edu

G. Arce (✉)
Department of Orthopaedic Surgery, Insituto Argentino de Diagnostico y Tratamiento, Marcelo T. de Alvear 2400, 1122, Buenos Aires, Argentina
e-mail: guillermorarce@ciudad.com.ar

appropriately powered study conclusions. In order to achieve this, universal classification systems and outcome assessment tools will be necessary.

This past year, a group was formed by members of the ISAKOS Arthroscopy Committee and the Upper Extremity Committee to standardize terminology for shoulder instability and rotator cuff disorders. These topics were chosen because over 80% of the presentations at the ISAKOS Meetings in Florence, Osaka, and Rio di Janeiro were related to one of these two conditions. The group has been led by Guillermo Arce and Kevin Shea. Other members include Klaus Bak, Mark Ferguson, Eiji Itoi, Emilio Calvo, Benno Ejnisman, Raffy Mirzayan, Ben Kibler, Jaap Willems, Augustus (Gus) Mazzocca, Matthew Provencher, Felix (Buddy) Savoie, and Philippe Hardy. Discussions took place via internet for a year and then a consensus meeting was held in February 2012 in San Francisco, CA, USA. The group strongly felt that in order to compare any research on one of these shoulder injuries, we would need a single system to classify injuries and a single outcome measure to report our results. The classification system should be already in use, if possible, validated for reliability, and easily used by physicians and researchers. Similarly, the outcome scores should be validated, already in use, and include both patient-completed measures and objective data.

The group first discussed the current systems used to classify rotator cuff tears. There was an agreement that a new system was needed to classify rotator cuff tears. These systems are critically reviewed by Paulo Belangero, Benno Ejnisman, and Guillermo Arce. The recommendation for a new ISAKOS System for Rotator Cuff Tears is presented by Emilio Calvo, who was the primary developer of this system.

We then reviewed all of the systems currently used to classify shoulder instability and concluded that a new system was necessary. The current systems are critically reviewed and a modification of the FEDS system is presented by Kevin Shea.

Lastly, we evaluated the current systems already in use to report the outcomes of treatment of shoulder instability and rotator cuff disease treatment. This review and our group consensus is presented by Guillermo Arce and Kevin Shea.

The goal of our work has been to present the idea that we all should use one scoring system to classify and report outcomes on every condition that we treat. In that way, we can review, compare, and pool our results in order to arrive at the best outcomes for our patients. These recommendations still need to be validated and will likely be improved by others with time. However, we believe that these recommendations are a good start in achieving our goals.

A Review of Rotator Cuff Classifications in Current Use

2

Paulo Santoro Belangero, Benno Ejnisman and Guillermo Arce

2.1 Background

To better understand the natural history of rotator cuff disease and its treatment, it is crucial to find a reliable method of classifying or describing rotator cuff tears. We can then use this classification to identify appropriate treatments for each type of tear that lead to the best outcomes. There are many rotator cuff classification systems in use today, making it difficult to compare results and to agree on proper treatment. In addition, when using any system, surgeons may not always agree on how a particular tear is classified.

After a comprehensive search in the literature available, Kuhn et al. were able to identify nine rotator cuff tear classifications systems that have been recommended to describe partial and full-thickness rotator cuff tears [1]. Each of these systems has been used in studying the outcomes of various treatments for rotator cuff tears. They developed a reliability study of 5 classification's systems: DeOrio (1984), Ellman (1995), Harryman (1991), Patte (1990), and Wolfgang (1974) [2–6]. The results from

---

P. S. Belangero (✉)
Federal University of Sao Paulo, Estado de Israel 435 Ap131, São Paulo,
SP 04022-001, Brazil
e-mail: psbelangero@gmail.com

B. Ejnisman
CETE-UNIFESP-EPM, Rua Vanderley 466 Ap232, São Paulo,
SP 5011001, Brazil
e-mail: bennoale@uol.com.br

G. Arce
Department of Orthopaedic Surgery, Insituto Argentino de Diagnostico y Tratamiento,
Marcelo T. de Alvear 2400, 1122 Buenos Aires, Argentina
e-mail: guillermorarce@ciudad.com.ar

that study demonstrated that experienced clinicians show very high agreement when deciding whether a rotator cuff tear is a partial-thickness tear or a full-thickness tear. In addition, clinicians are adept at agreeing on the side involved (articular or bursal) when a partial-thickness tear is identified. However, clinicians could not agree on the depth of the partial-thickness tears [1]. With regard to full-thickness tears, the results suggested that none of the classification systems resulted in excellent agreement [1].

Many factors as size, shape, retraction and fatty infiltration, are now recognized as being important in the preoperative assessment of the patient with a symptomatic rotator cuff tear. These factors are necessary to dictate appropriate surgical treatment and to counsel the patient on realistic expectations of postoperative outcome [7]. Any universal classification system should include these factors.

Most of the classifications systems in use today were developed for either for full or partial thickness tears. The first step in deciding on a universal classification system is to critically review each of these systems.

2.2 Partial-Thickness Tears Classifications

Ellman [8] was the first to popularize a system to classify partial thickness tears based on intra-operative findings. In his system, a Grade 1 tear is <3 mm deep, a Grade 2 is tear 3–6 mm in depth but not exceeding one-half of the tendon thickness and a Grade 3 tear >6 mm deep. Others have simplified the system referring to 6 mm or less (<50 %) or >6 mm (greater than 50 %). While there are not any studies on reliability, this system is used by many to decide on the type of surgical treatment. Snyder [9] included a more detailed classification of partial tears in his system (see below). His system has not been validated for reliability. Neither system includes interstitial tears that do not communicate with either the articular of bursal surfaces.

More recently, Habermeyer et al. have developed a new arthroscopic classification of articular-sided supraspinatus footprint lesions and a prospective comparison with Snyder's and Ellman's classification [10, 11]. They realized that, neither the classification of Snyder nor that of Ellman reproduced the extension of the partial-thickness rotator cuff tear in the transverse and coronal planes related to its etiologic pathomorphology [11]. Their system includes a gradation of the thickness of the partial articular-side tear as does Ellman and Snyder (see Fig. 2.1). It also includes a classification of tear size and location in the sagittal plane (see Fig. 2.2).

Although this system seems to be more complete than the previous, its still is an arthroscopic classification, which limits its use. It has not been validated for reliability and does not include a classification of bursal-side or interstitial tears.

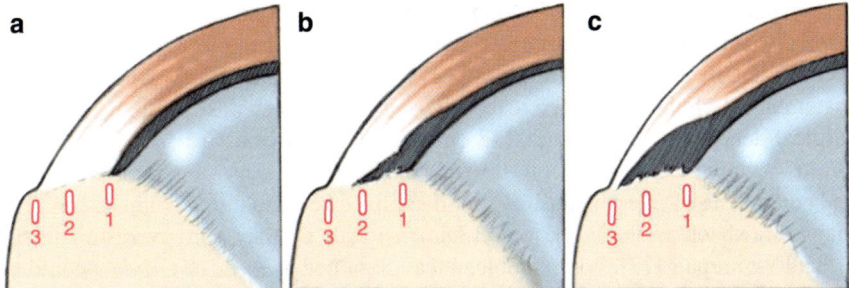

Fig. 2.1 The Habermayer classification of partial tears in the coronal plane. Longitudinal extension of articular-sided supraspinatus tendon tears in coronal plane. **a** Type 1 tear: small tear within transition zone from cartilage to bone. **b** Type 2 tear: extension of tear up to center of footprint. **c** Type 3 tear: extension of tear up to greater tuberosity (Reprinted with permission)

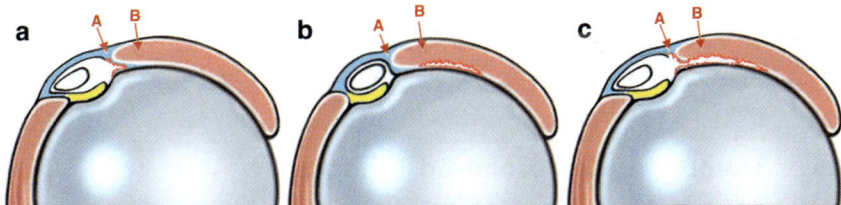

Fig. 2.2 Habermayer classification of partial tears in the sagittal plane. Sagittal extension of articular-sided supraspinatus tendon tears in transverse plane. **a** Type A tear: tear of coracohumeral ligament continuing into medial border of supraspinatus tendon. **b** Type B tear: isolated tear within crescent zone. **c** Type C tear: tear extending from lateral border of pulley system over medial border of supraspinatus tendon up to area of crescent zone (Reprinted with permission)

2.3 Full-Thickness Tear Classification Systems

Today, many factors are felt to be important in describing full-thickness rotator cuff tears. These include: size, number of tendons involved, tear shape tissue quality, and CT/MRI assessment of fatty infiltration and atrophy of the muscles attached to the torn tendons. In a review of the commonly used systems, not one included all of these factors.

2.4 Tear Size

One of the most commonly used classification systems was developed by DeOrio and Cofield [2]. They classified tears by the anterior-posterior length of the tendon that was torn off of the humeral head as measured at the time of surgery. The system classified tears as *small* if the tear was less than one cm, *medium* if the tear was between 1 and 3 cm, *large* 3–5 cm, and *massive* if the tear was greater than 5 cm in length. Bayne and Bateman [12] used a similar, but less commonly used system in which they classified tears as *Grade 1* if the tear was less than 1 cm after surgical debridement, *Grade 2*: 1–3 cm after debridement, *Grade 3*: 3–5 cm and *Grade 4*: global tear, no cuff left. It would appear that the classifications are similar and could be used interchangeably, but there have been no direct comparisons. The major drawback is these are not 3-Dimensional, so they can overestimate the difficulty of repair [13]. For example, a tear classified as *large* or *Grade 3* could be a 4 cm tear with minimal retraction and healthy, robust tissue, or a 4 cm tear retracted to the labrum with thin, friable tissue. In addition, they do not identify which tendon(s) are involved. Most surgeons would agree that a repair 2 cm tear of the supraspinatus may have a very different outcome when compared to a 2 cm tear of the subscapularis. These classifications do not normalized to the patient's size, so the value of the absolute size of the rotator cuff tear remains in question [1]. Finally, important factors related to surgical procedures as tear shape and fatty infiltration are not included. Nevertheless, the DeOrio and Cofield classification is one of the two most systems most commonly used in the orthopaedic literature.

2.5 Number of Compromised Tendons

Harryman [4] developed a classification system based on the number of tendons involved in the tear identified at the time of surgery. Stage 1A is a partial thickness tear, Stage 1B is a full-thickness tear isolated to the supraspinatus. Stage II includes the supraspinatus and at a portion of the infraspinatus. Stage III includes the entire supraspinatus, the infraspinatus and the subscapularis tendons. Stage IV is rotator cuff arthropathy. This system has not been validated.

Classifications systems based in the number of tendons involved as Harryman's [4] are important predicting the extent of surgical procedure necessary to repair the tear [14], but do not differentiate the tear pattern or method of repair [13].

2.6 Tear Shape

Ellman and Gartsman [3] developed a classification system to take into account the three dimensional nature of rotator cuff tears. *Crescent-shaped* tears are wide (anterior-posterior) with minimal retraction. *Reverse-L* and *L-shaped* tears have some portion of the tendon torn off of the humeral head and then extend into the tendon medially forming the shape of the letter L or a backwards L. The medial-lateral tear often is through the rotator interval between the subscapularis and supraspinatus, or in the interval between the supraspinatus and infraspinatus. *Trapezoidal* tears are larger looking like a trapezoid and *Massive* tears are larger and irreparable. The classification, like the previous ones, is based on the findings at the time of surgery. It has not been validated.

One large drawback to each of the systems described above is the inability to use them pre-operatively to give the patient a prognosis for a successful outcome. The ideal classification system, once validated, should not only describe and categorize tear patterns, but it should also eventually be used to predict the type of surgery necessary to repair the tear and give a patient an idea of the eventual outcome of the surgical procedure. Because these systems classify the tear only during surgery, they cannot be used to prognostic purposes. We are not aware of any study that applies these classifications to pre-operative imaging.

Burkhart [13] developed a geometric classification system based on pre-operative MRI imaging. He classified the tear pattern into 4 shapes and felt that this shape was correlated to outcome. Measuring the tear on both sagittal and coronal MRI images, *Type 1* tears are crescent-shaped tears that are relatively short in the coronal image and wide on the sagittal image. *Type 2* tears are longitudinal (U-shaped and L-shaped) tears that are relatively long on the coronal and short on the sagittal images. *Type 3* tears are massive and contracted tears being both long on the coronal and wide on the sagittal images. Type 4 tears include a massive tear and glenohumeral arthrosis and loss of acromiohumeral distance indicative of rotator cuff arthropathy. The advantage of this system is that it is used pre-operatively.

These classifications rely in tear exclusively configuration alone. Although they add information that can help the surgical preparation (and prognosis in Burkhart's), they lack information about size, retraction and tendon quality.

2.7 Others (Complete/Complex)

Patte [5] developed a system that incorporated several factors including: (1) Extent of the rotator cuff tears; (2) Topography of the tear in sagittal plane; (3) Topography of the tear in frontal plane; (4) Topography quality of the muscles of the torn tendons; and (5) State of the long head of the biceps as measured on pre-operative imaging. Patte's classification is divided in 5 main categories and which one of then is further separated in many items. The most commonly used portion of the classification is retraction of the supraspinatus tendon in the coronal plane as shown below. Stage I is a tear with minimal retraction, Stage II is a tear retracted medial to the humeral head footprint but not to the glenoid, and Stage III is a tear retracted to the level of the glenoid (Fig. 2.3).

The Patte classification has been found to have consistently moderate agreement in assessing tear retraction in various studies [1, 15]. It has also been shown to have some prognostic value after rotator cuff repair [18]. However, size, shape and tissue quality as well as differentiation of the tendons involved are not included.

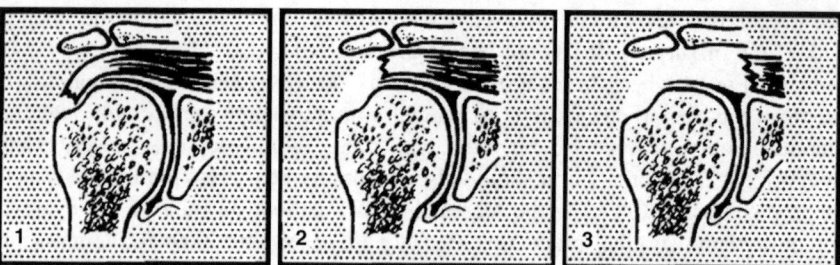

Fig. 2.3 Patte classification of rotator cuff tears. The Patte score assesses the degree of tendon retraction in the frontal plane on MRI: full-thickness tear with little tendon retraction (*1*), retraction of tendon to level of humeral head (*2*), and retraction of tendon to level of glenoid (*3*) (Reprinted with permission)

Snyder [9] developed a comprehensive classification to describe the extent of the tear, the location and the size. The location of the tear is classified as *Articular*, *Bursal*, or *Complete* thickness tears. Partial Thickness Tears are subclassified as 0—normal, 1—minimal superficial bursal or synovial irritation or slight capsular fraying over a small area, 2—Fraying and failure of some rotator cuff fibers in addition to synovial bursal or capsular injury, 3—More severe rotator cuff injury fraying and fragmentation of tendon fibers often involving the whole of a cuff tendon, usually <3 cm or 4—Very severe partial rotator cuff tear that contains a sizeable flap tear and more than one tendon. These descriptions are more qualitative than quantitative and do not have adequate inter-observer agreement.

Full Thickness tears are classified as: C1—Small complete tear, pinhole sized, C2—Moderate tear <2 cm of only one tendon without retraction, C3—Large complete tear with an entire tendon with minimal retraction usually 3–4 cm, C4—Massive rotator cuff tear involving 2 or more rotator cuff tendon with associated retraction and scarring of the remaining tendon. This system, as the others does not include all of the factors felt to be important in fully classifying tears of the rotator cuff tendons.

It is clear that the more complex the system, the less likely the agreement will be; on the other hand, a good classification should give solid information about type of surgery, difficulties and prognosis.

2.8 Tendon Quality

It has been shown that repair integrity is related to preoperative tear size and fatty infiltration on preoperative magnetic resonance imaging (MRI) [16, 17]. It has also been shown that fatty infiltration and muscle atrophy do not improve after successful structural repair of the rotator cuff and their presence correlates with poor

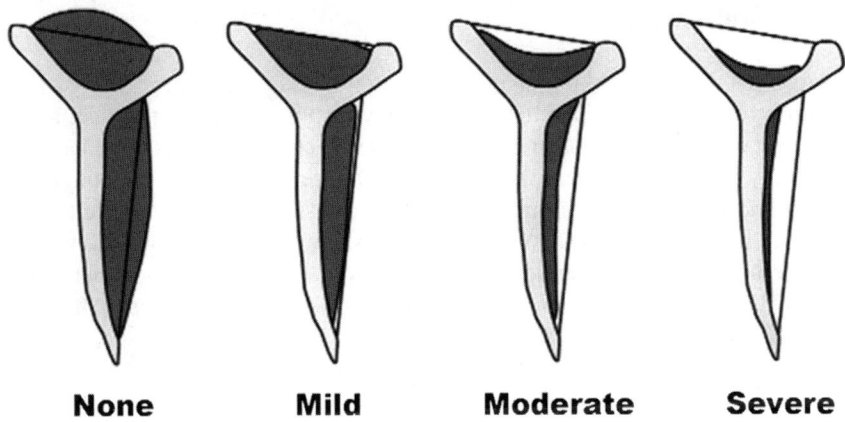

Fig. 2.4 Warner classification of rotator cuff atrophy. The Warner grading of muscle atrophy is based on the relation of the muscle to a straight line connecting either the coracoid to the scapular spine (assessing the supraspinatus) or the coracoid to the tip of the scapula (assessing the infraspinatus) (Reprinted with permission)

functional outcomes [18, 19]. Thus, a complete rotator cuff classification system should include information about the pre-operative muscle atrophy and fatty infiltration of the rotator cuff muscles.

Thomazeau [10] classified the supraspinatus muscle belly based on the occupation ratio in the supraspinatus fossa in T1-weighted oblique-sagittal images (MRI). Stage I was normal or slightly atrophied, Stage II showed moderate atrophy, and Stage III was serious or severe atrophy. Warner et al. described a grading scale for muscle atrophy based on the oblique sagittal-plane magnetic resonance images [6] (see Fig. 2.4).

The system grades the atrophy of either the supraspinatus or infraspinatus muscle belly as none, mild, moderate or severe. Studies have shown moderate inter-observer agreement using this classification [6]. Atrophy if the infraspinatus has been shown to correlate with outcome in at least one study [18].

Goutallier introduced a classification of fatty infiltration of the supraspinatus based on the presence of fatty streaks within the muscle belly using CT images; Stage 0 is normal muscle, Stage I: muscle with some fatty streaks, Stage II: fatty infiltration is important, but there still more muscle than fat, Stage III: there is as much fat as muscle and Stage IV: more fat than muscle is present. This classification system is often quoted but studies have not shown good inter-observer agreement [6] and have not, as of yet been correlated to outcome. Fuchs has published a similar classification using MRI.

2.9 Conclusion

A surgeon's decision-making algorithm is often based on evidence derived from outcome studies. To appropriately apply study results to clinical practice, a reliance on standardized patient study populations is necessary. This is often based on commonly used classification schemes [7]. Our review has not identified any classification system in current use that includes all of the factors felt to be important in classifying rotator cuff tear patterns. Thus, a new system that includes tear size, location, shape, retraction, location and tissue quality that displays high inter and intra-observer reliability is necessary. (Please see references [20, 21] at the end of the chapter.)

References

1. Kuhn JE, Dunn WR, Ma B et al (2007) Interobserver agreement in the classification of rotator cuff tears. Am J Sports Med 35:437–441
2. DeOrio JK, Cofield RH (1984) Results of a second attempt at surgical repair of a failed initial rotator cuff repair. J Bone Joint Surg Am 66:563–567
3. Ellman H (1993) Rotator cuff disorders. In: Ellman H, Gartsman GM (eds) Arthroscopic shoulder surgery and related disorders. Lea and Febiger, Philadelphia, pp 98–119
4. Harryman DT, Mack LA, Wang K, Jackins SE, Richardson ML, Matsen FA (1991) Repairs of the rotator cuff. Correlation of functional results with integrity of the cuff. J Bone Joint Surg Am 73:982–989
5. Patte D (1990) Classification of rotator cuff lesions. Clin Orthop Relat Res 254:81–86
6. Wolfgang GL (1974) Surgical repairs of tears of the rotator cuff of the shoulder. J Bone Joint Surg Am 56:14–26
7. Lippe J, Spang JT, Leger RR, Arciero RA, Mazzocca AD, Shea KP (2012) Inter-rater agreement of the Goutallier, Patte, and Warner classification scores using preoperative magnetic resonance imaging in patients with rotator cuff tears. Arthrosc: J Arthrosc Relat Surg 28(2)(February):154–159
8. Ellman H (1990) Diagnosis and treatment of incomplete rotator cuff tears. Clin Orthop Relat Res 254:64–74
9. Snyder SJ (2003) Arthroscopic classification of rotator cuff lesions and surgical decision making. In: Snyder SJ (ed) Shoulder arthroscopy. Lippincott Williams & Wilkins, Philadelphia, pp 201–207
10. Habermeyer P, Magosch P, Lichtenberg S (2006) Classifications of rotator cuff. In: Walch G, Boileau P (eds) Classifications and scores of the shoulder. Springer, Berlin
11. Habermeyer P, Krieter MC, Tang K-L, Lichtenberg S, Magosch P (2008) A new arthroscopic classification of articular-sided supraspinatus footprint lesions: a prospective comparison with Snyder's and Ellman's classification. J Shoulder Elbow Surg (Nov–Dec) 17(6):909–913
12. Bayne O, Bateman J (1984) Long-term results of surgical repair of full-thickness rotator cuff tears. In: Bateman JE, Welsh R (eds) Surgery of the shoulder. CV Mosby, Philadelphia, pp 167–171
13. Davidson J, Burkhart SS (2010) The geometric classification of rotator cuff tears: a system linking tear pattern to treatment and prognosis. Arthroscopy 26:417–424
14. Nho SJ, Brown BS, Lyman S, Adler RS, Altchek DW, MacGillivray JD (2009) Prospective analysis of arthroscopic rotator cuff repair: prognostic factors affecting clinical and ultrasound outcome. J Shoulder Elbow Surg (Jan–Feb 2009) 18(1):13–20. Epub: 16 Sept 2008

15. Spencer EE, Dunn WR, Wright RW et al (2008) Interobserver agreement in the classification of rotator cuff tears using magnetic resonance imaging. Am J Sports Med 36:99–103
16. Goutallier D, Postel JM, Bernageau J, Lavau L, Voisin MC (1994) Fatty muscle degeneration in cuff ruptures. Pre- and postoperative evaluation by CT scan. Clin Orthop Relat Res 304:78–83
17. Oh JH, Kim SH, Ji HM, Jo KH, Bin SW, Gong HS (2009) Prognostic factors affecting anatomic outcome of rotator cuff repair and correlation with functional outcome. Arthroscopy 25:30–39
18. Gladstone JN, Bishop JY, Lo IK, Flatow EL (2007) Fatty infiltration and atrophy of the rotator cuff do not improve after rotator cuff repair and correlate with poor functional outcome. Am J Sports Med 35:719–728
19. Melis B, Nemoz C, Walch G (2009) Muscle fatty infiltration in rotator cuff tears: Descriptive analysis of 1688 cases. Orthop Traumatol Surg Res 95:319–324
20. Fuchs B, Weishaupt D, Zanetti M, Hodler J, Gerber C (1999) Fatty degeneration of the muscles of the rotator cuff: assessment by computed tomography versus magnetic resonance imaging. J Shoulder Elbow Surg 8:599–605
21. Warner JJP, Higgins L, Parsons IM IV, Dowdy P (2001) Diagnosis and treatment of anterosuperior rotator cuff tears. J Shoulder Elbow Surg 10:37–46

ISAKOS Classification System for Rotator Cuff Tears

Emilio Calvo and the ISAKOS Upper Extremity and Anthroscopy Committees

3.1 Introduction

Many classification systems have been used to describe rotator cuff tears in the worldwide orthopaedic literature. However, there is not one current standard classification that includes all the types of rotator cuff tears, describes its key characteristics or is universally utilized.

As in other orthopaedic conditions, any classification for rotator cuff tears should follow several principles. First, the classification system should be already in use, if possible, validated for reliability, and easily used by physicians and researchers. We are aware in the orthopaedic literature of failed attempts of new classifications aimed to overcome the limitations of their classic counterparts simply because the orthopaedic community is used to the "classical language" (i.e. new classifications of proximal humeral fractures to substitute the classical Neer-Codman classification). Second, it should be descriptive to define the location and anatomy of the tear, helping all surgeons to understand precisely its characteristics. Third, the classification should be useful to dictate appropriate treatment in each specific case, and fourth, it should also have a predictive value both to guide physicians and to transmit the patient realistic expectations of postoperative outcome. Finally, the orthopaedic literature is full of classifications that, although addressing the details of the specific problem, are difficult to remember. This represents a significant limitation to facilitate its use, and the classification for

---

ISAKOS Upper Extremity and Anthroscopy Committee: Emilio Calvo, Kevin Shea, Benno Ejnisman, Guillermo Arce, W. Ben Kibler, Felix Savoie III, Alberto Pochini, Eiji Itoi, Hiroyuki Sugaya, Giovanni Di Giacomo, Yon Sik Yoo, Dan Guttmann, Tom Ludvigsen, Augustus Mazzocca, Gregory Bain, John Uribe, Matthew Provencher, Jaap Willems, Francisco Vergara

E. Calvo and the ISAKOS Upper Extremity and Anthroscopy Committees (✉)
Shoulder and Elbow Reconstructive Surgery Unit, Department of Orthopedic Surgery, Fundacion Jimenez Diaz—Capio, Av. Reyes Catolicos 2, 28040, Madrid, Spain
e-mail: ecalvo@fjd.es; emilio.calvo@fmail.com

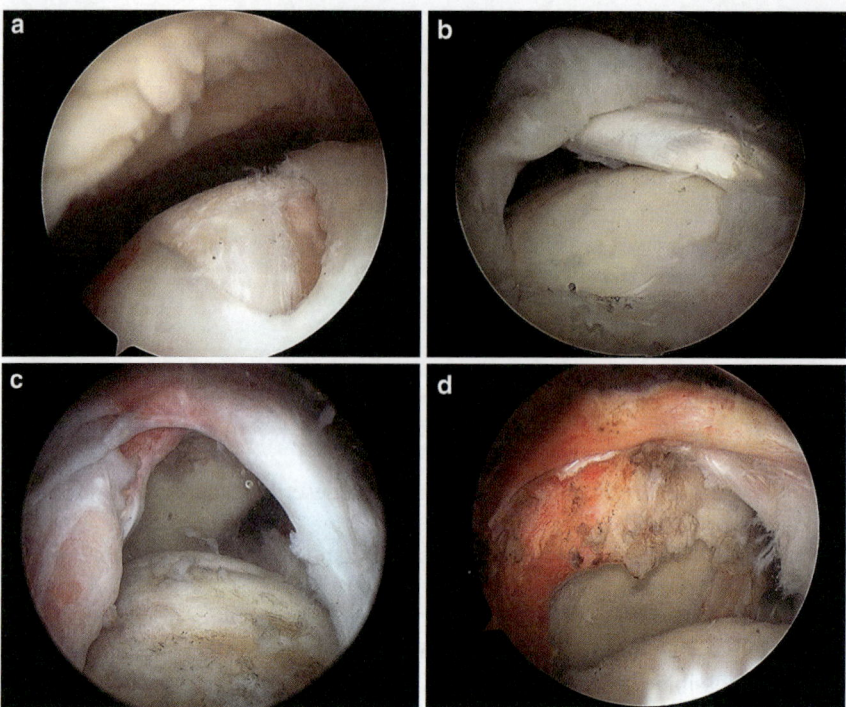

Fig. 3.1 Arthroscopic views of full thickness rotator cuff tears from the bursal side. **a** small C1; **b** moderate C2; **c** large C3; **d** massive C4

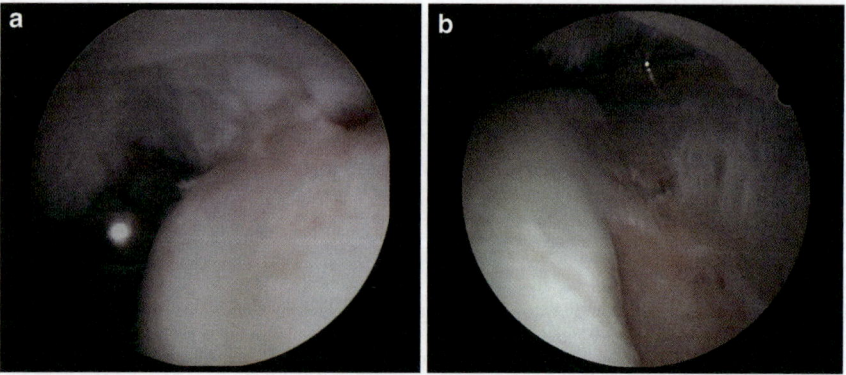

Fig. 3.2 Arthroscopic views of partial articular sided supraspinatus tears involving fewer (**a**) and over 50 % (**b**) of tendon thickness

rotator cuff must be not only ready to be understood, but also easy to remember and follow. Acronyms can be helpful in this sense (Figs. 3.1, 3.2, 3.3, 3.4, 3.5).

After reviewing the available rotator cuff scoring's systems, the ISAKOS Shoulder Terminology Group has developed a new system. The ISAKOS grading system is a complete and straightforward method to describe all rotator cuff tears. It relies on the fact that a good system should allow the surgeon to predict difficulties during the procedure and advise about prognostics. It is comprehensive and user-friendly. This system is explained below, and encompasses five essentials characteristics with regards to tears: pattern (P), extension (E), fatty atrophy (A), retraction(R), and location (L), conforming the acronym "PEARL" (Table 3.1).

3.2 Location

Most classifications reported in the literature have been suggested to describe posterosuperior rotator cuff tears involving the supraspinatus, infraspinatus and teres minor, but only recently subscapularis tears have drawn some attention. Since the characteristics as well as therapeutic and prognostic implications of posterosuperior and anterior rotator cuff tears are often different, we suggest defining first the anatomic location of the rotator cuff tear, posterosuperior or anterior.

3.3 Extension

Traditionally, rotator cuff tears have been described as partial or full thickness.

Classification systems for full-thickness posterosuperior tears have been based on the size of the tear or the number of tendons involved [1–3]. The information on the extension of the tear, either given as area or number of tendons involved, is important predicting the extent of surgical procedure and soft tissue releases necessary to repair it. However, the classifications based on the size of the tear must be bidimensional since a unidimensional description, as suggested by DeOrio and Cofield, can be misleading because it measures the tear size only anterior to posterior. A complete cuff avulsion described as massive, implying a difficult repair and unfavorable prognosis, may in fact lie directly over the bed of the insertion site, be easy to repair, and have a predictably good result [1]. For these reasons we suggest following the classification system of posterosuperior rotator cuff tears suggested by Snyder [4].The system described by Snyder provides information not only on the size, but also on the number of tendons involved and the degree of scarring. Full thickness tears are classified as C1 (small complete tear, pinhole sized), C2 (moderate tear less than 2 cm of only one tendon without retraction), C3 (large complete tear with an entire tendon with minimal retraction usually 3–4 cm), or C4 (massive rotator cuff tear involving 2 or more rotator cuff tendon with associated retraction and scarring of the remaining tendon) (Sect. 3. 1).

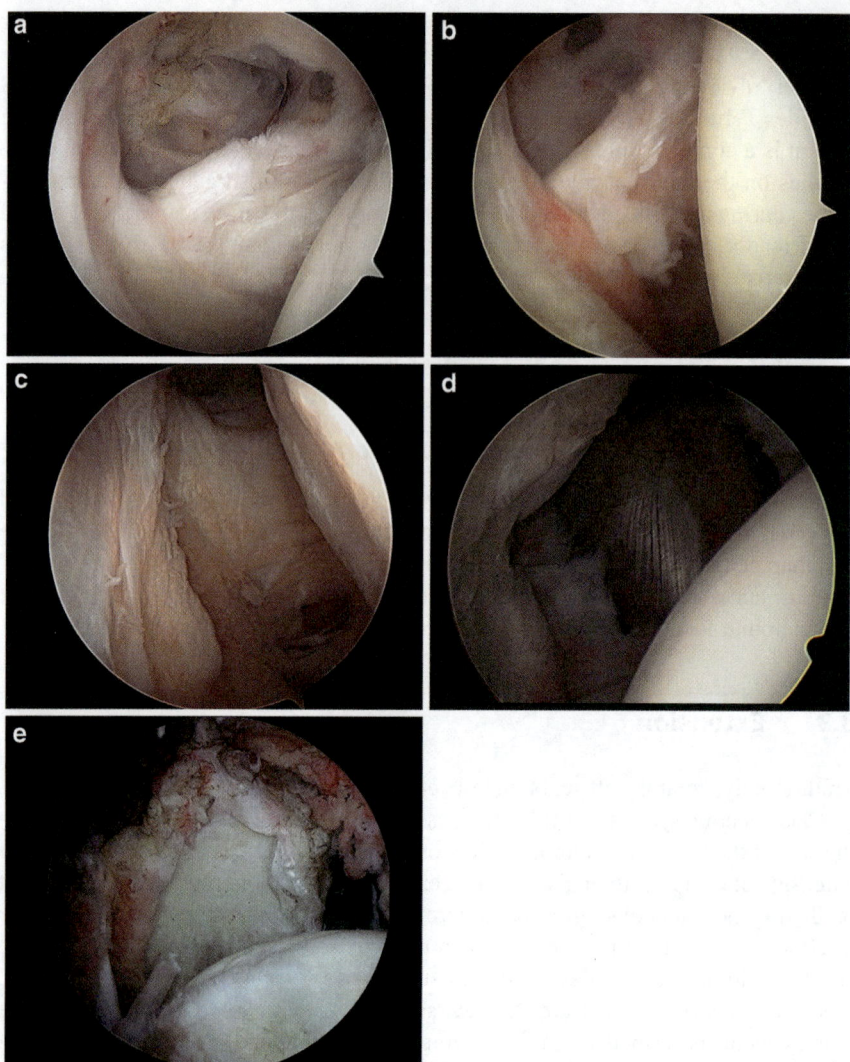

Fig. 3.3 Types of subscapularis tendon tears. **a** Tendon fraying at the superior edge; **b** partial detachment of the superior tendon third; **c** full tendon avulsion with inferior muscle attachment preservation; **d** complete subscapularis detachment, humeral head is cantered, no signs of glenohumeral arthropaty are observed; **e** massive rotator cuff tear involving full subscapularis rupture, and superior migration of the humeral head

With regard to partial thickness rotator cuff tears, experimental and clinical studies have demonstrated that tears involving more than half of the tendon thickness are a significant to threat tendon integrity, and that they outperform

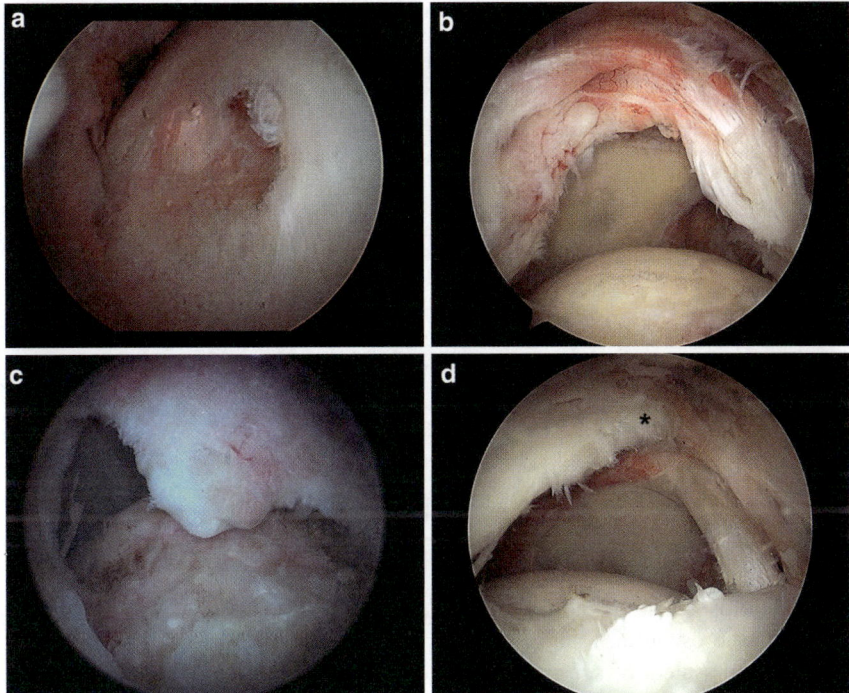

Fig. 3.4 Geometric classification of rotator cuff tears. **a** Small crescent shape tear; **b** U-shaped tear; **c** L-shaped tear; **d** reverse L-shaped tear

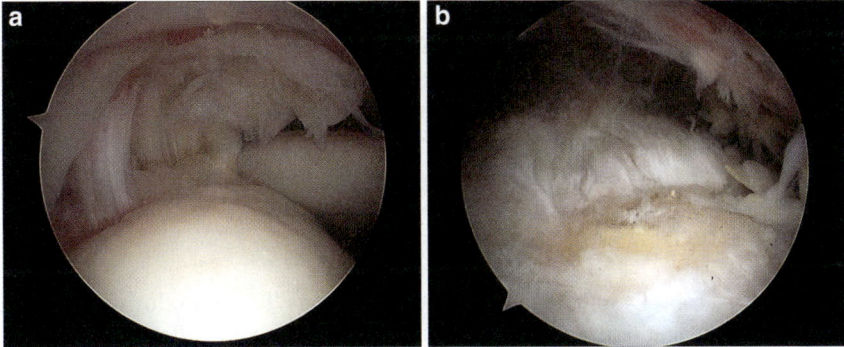

Fig. 3.5 Arthroscopic views of partial thickness supraspinatus tears involving different aspects of the tendon. **a** Articular-side tear; **b** bursal-side tear

better if treated surgically [5, 6]. Based on these observations we recommend in partial thickness rotator cuff tears to define the site and tendon tissue involvement as over or fewer than 50 % of tendon thickness (Sect. 3.2).

Table 3.1 ISAKOS Rotator cuff tear classification system

Location (L)	Extension (E)	Pattern (P)	Fatty atrophy (A)[a]		Retraction (R)
Partial thickness posterosuperior	>50 % thickness <50 % thickness	A (Articular) B (Bursal) I (Interstitial)	SS0 SS1 SS2	IS0 IS1 IS2	
Full thickness Postero-superior (SS-IS)	C1 C2 C3 C4 (Massive)	C U L rL (reverse L)	SS3 SS4	IS3 IS4	1 2 3
Anterior (SC)	1 2 3 4 5		SC0 SC1 SC2 SC3 SC4		

[a] *SS* supraspinatus, *IS* infraspinatus, *SC* subscapularis

The etiology, pattern, surgical approach of subscapularis tear is different from those of posterosuperior rotator cuff tears. Lafosse et al. put forward extensively a classification system of subscapularis tears that shows the pattern and the size of five different stages based on anatomic observations with arthroscopy, and showed also the surgical approach for its reconstruction [7] (Sect. 3.3).Type 1 lesions are simple erosions of the superior third, without bone avulsion. Type 2 consists of detachment restricted to the superior third. Type 3 involves the entire height of the tendon insertion, but without muscular detachment of the inferior third, with limited tendon retraction. Type 4 is complete subscapularis detachment from the lesser tuberosity of the humerus, but with the humeral head remaining well centered, without contact with the coracoid on internal rotation on CT-scan. Type 5 also represents complete rupture, but with anterosuperior migration of the humeral head, which comes into contact with the coracoid, with associated fatty infiltration.

3.4 Pattern

The systems for classification of rotator cuff tears based exclusively on the extension of the tear or the number of tendons involved do not differentiate specific tear pattern or method of repair. Davidson and Burkhart described a three-dimensional geometric classification obtained from preoperative magnetic resonance imaging (MRI) or at arthroscopy that helps orthopaedic surgeons communicate about tears of the supraspinatus, infraspinatus, and teres minor based on tear pattern recognition, and furnishes important guidance on the treatment technique and prognosis for each tear type [8]. This geometric classification defines four different patterns: crescent-shaped tears, U-shaped tears, L-shaped tears, and reverse L-shaped tears (Sect. 3. 4). Crescent-shaped tears are relatively short in the coronal image and wide on the sagittal image. They are commonly mobile from medial to lateral and can usually be repaired by fixing the tendon end directly to the footprint on the greater humeral tuberosity. U-shaped and L-shaped tears are relatively long on the coronal and short on the sagittal images. These tears are usually mobile in an anteroposterior direction and frequently must be repaired by a side-to-side or margin convergence technique. The advantage of this system is that it can be used pre- and intraoperatively.

For partial thickness rotator cuff tears the classification scheme proposed by Ellman that included specific considerations of the site of the tear along the tendon thickness (articular surface, bursal surface, or intratendinous) is suggested [9] (Sect. 3. 5).

3.5 Atrophy

Tear size and tendon retraction, fatty infiltration and muscle atrophy are major prognostic factors of the structural and functional outcomes after rotator cuff tear repair [10].Thus, a complete rotator cuff classification system should include information about the pre-operative muscle status. Goutallier et al. first described a classification of fatty infiltration of the supraspinatus based on the presence of fatty streaks within the muscle belly using CT images, and later Fuchs et al. validated the same system to be used with MRI images [11, 12]. The classification defines five degrees of muscle fatty infiltration that can be ascribed to all the four rotator cuff muscles (Grade 0 = Normal muscle, grade 1 = some fatty streaks, grade 2 = less than 50 % fatty muscle atrophy, i.e. more muscle than fat, grade 3 = 50 % fatty muscle atrophy, i.e. equal muscle and fat, and grade 4 = more than 50 % muscle atrophy, i.e. more fat than muscle).

3.6 Retraction

Tendon retraction is a common phenomenon in rotator cuff tears, and it has been shown that formation of a recurrent tendon defect correlates with the timing of tendon retraction; and clinical outcome correlates with its magnitude [13, 14]. The most commonly used portion of the classification is retraction of the supraspinatus tendon in the coronal plane shown in imaging studies as described by Patte (stage 1 = tear with minimal retraction, stage 2 = tear retracted medial to the humeral head footprint but not to the glenoid, and stage 3 = tear retracted to the level of the glenoid. In addition, it is recommended to test tendon retraction intraoperatively to establish a surgical strategy defining the soft tissue releases and slides to be performed, and to assist in the prediction of the final outcome of the repair [15].

3.7 Conclusions

The ISAKOS Upper Limb and Arthroscopy Committees believe that the presented classification system for rotator cuff tears combine the important factors from those classifications in current use into on unified evaluation system easy to remember that fulfil the needs of the surgeons to better classify the rotator cuff tears. Compared to the previous classifications, this new system has advantages. It is fitted for both posterosuperior and subscapularis tears and for partial or full thickness tears, gives details on the size and geographic patterns of the tears useful to establish an appropriate treatment, while providing relevant information on the prognosis of the repair based not only on the size, but also on tendon retraction and the muscle atrophy and fatty infiltration.

References

1. DeOrio JK, Cofield RH (1984) Results of a second attempt at surgical repair of a failed initial rotator cuff repair. J Bone Joint Surg Am 66:563–567
2. Harryman DT, Mack LA, Wang K, Jackins SE, Richardson ML, Matsen FA (1991) Repairs of the rotator cuff. Correlation of functional results with integrity of the cuff. J Bone Joint Surg Am 73:982–989
3. Gerber C, Fuchs B, Hodler J (2000) The results of repair of massive tears of the rotator cuff. J Bone Joint Surg Am 82:505–515
4. Snyder SJ (2003) Arthroscopic classification of rotator cuff lesions and surgical decision-making. In: Snyder SJ (ed) Shoulder Arthroscopy. Lippincott Williams & Wilkins, Philadelphia, pp 201–207
5. Weber SC (1999) Arthroscopic debridement and acromioplasty versus mini-open repair in the treatment of significant partial-thickness rotator cuff tears. Arthroscopy 15:126–131
6. Sano H, Wakabayashi I, Itoi E (2006) Stress distribution in the supraspinatus tendon with partial-thickness tears: an analysis using two-dimensional finite element model. J Shoulder Elbow Surg 15:100–105
7. Lafosse L, Jost B, Reiland Y, Audebert S, Toussaint B, Gobezie R (2007) Structural integrity and clinical outcomes after arthroscopic repair of isolated subscapularis tears. J Bone Joint Surg Am 89:1184–1193
8. Davidson J, Burkhart SS (2010) The geometric classification of rotator cuff tears: a system linking tear pattern to treatment and prognosis. Arthroscopy 26:417–424
9. Ellman H (1990) Diagnosis and treatment of incomplete rotator cuff tears. Clin Orthop Relat Res 254:64–74
10. Oh JH, Kim SH, Ji HM, Jo KH, Bin SW, Gong HS (2009) Prognostic factors affecting anatomic outcome of rotator cuff repair and correlation with functional outcome. Arthroscopy 25:30–39
11. Goutallier D, Postel JM, Bernageau J, Lavau L, Voisin MC (1994) Fatty muscle degeneration in cuff ruptures. Pre- and postoperative evaluation by CT scan. Clin Orthop Relat Res 304:78–83

12. Fuchs B, Weishaupt D, Zanetti M, Hodler J, Gerber C (1999) Fatty degeneration of the muscles of the rotator cuff: assessment by computed tomography versus magnetic resonance imaging. J Shoulder Elbow Surg 8:599–605
13. McCarron JA, Derwin KA, Bey MJ, Polster JM, Schils JP, Ricchetti ET, Iannotti JP (2012) Failure with continuity in rotator cuff repair "healing". Am J Sports Med (Epub ahead of print)
14. Lippe J, Spang JT, Leger RR, Arciero RA, Mazzocca AD, Shea KP (2012) Inter-rater agreement of the Goutallier, Patte, and Warner classification scores using preoperative magnetic resonance imaging in patients with rotator cuff tears. Arthroscopy 28:154–159
15. Patte D (1990) Classification of rotator cuff lesions. Clin Orthop Relat Res 254:81–86

Review of Current Classifications of Shoulder Instability

Kevin P. Shea

4.1 Background

Classifying glenohumeral instability poses a significant challenge. Unlike the classification of fractures such as the AO classification of ankle fractures, or even soft-tissue injuries such as rotator cuff tears, glenohumeral instability constitutes a symptom not readily identified on an x-ray or MRI. Attempts to classify instability in the literature have actually contributed to ongoing confusion. The first reported classification was simple: anterior versus posterior instability. The physician relied on patient's account, radiographs if available, and a physical examination to determine the direction of the dislocation. Rowe et al. [1] and others [2] identified that the shoulder could be unstable but not dislocate and recurrent subluxations and "dead-arm" syndrome were added. The concept of multidirectional instability by Neer and Foster [3] added to the classification by noting that some patients could become unstable secondary to repetitive microtrauma or congenital shoulder laxity. They reported on that the sulcus sign was considered a vital component of this diagnosis. This report confirmed that not all shoulder instability was the result of a traumatic lesion, but its broad definition of multidirectional instability has led to conflicting reports in the literature [4].

K. P. Shea (✉)
University of Connecticut Health Center, Farmington Avenue 263, Farmington, CT 06034-4037, USA
e-mail: shea@uchc.edu

4.2 Various Classifications of Shoulder Instability

Matsen et al. [5] divided instability into 2 categories using the acronym TUBS (Traumatic, Unilateral instability that was associated with a Bankart lesion and usually required Surgery) and AMBRI (Atraumatic Multidirectional instability that was usually Bilateral and should be treated with Rehabilitation). These patients usually had a sulcus sign. While this classification was simple and did divide instability into traumatic and atraumatic, certainly did not cover individuals with shoulder laxity who have a traumatic dislocation. Further, there are many patients with a sulcus sign who do not have symptoms.

Gerber and Nyffeler [6] emphasized the importance of identifying the etiology at the onset of instability and the confusion in the literature between clinically measured laxity and symptomatic shoulder instability. In that study, the authors pointed out that laxity is a genetic trait that varies from person to person. They recognized that hyperlaxity could be a risk factor for developing late-onset instability through either a traumatic event or repetitive microtrauma. Finally, the authors affirmed that clinical examinations at the office setting or at the operating room could only document laxity (i.e. sulcus sign of increased anterior or posterior translation) and the diagnosis of instability. They developed a system of instability that included Static Instability, Dynamic Instability and Voluntary Instability. This classification system has been helpful to the understanding of instability, but does not completely classify all types.

Jobe et al. [7] reported on glenohumeral instability unique to the overhead and throwing athlete. Prior to his report, shoulder pain in these athletes was felt to be secondary to rotator cuff impingement. The authors suggested that athletes had impingement secondary to laxity developed due to repetitive overhead athletics; recommending shoulder stabilization to treat the symptoms in case rehabilitation failed.

Kuhn et al. [8, 9] performed a comprehensive review of the orthopaedic literature with regards to the classification of shoulder instability and concluded that no system could describe all shoulder instabilities. The authors stated that every system published so far was based on expert opinion and had not been validated. Furthermore, Kuhn et al. developed the FEDS system, an acronym that stands for Frequency of instability, Etiology of the instability, Direction of the instability, and Severity of the Instability. They eliminated the concept of multidirectional instability altogether, and instead relied on the patient report and physical examination to determine the direction with most symptoms. This system has been extensively tested for reliability and content validity and is the best system published to date.

However, Kuhn et al. eliminated the pain in the overhead athlete as it did not meet their definition of instability, pain and a feeling of looseness. While they make an excellent argument for exclusion of these patients' subgroup, many surgeons continue to believe that pain in the overhead athlete should be recognized as instability. In addition, voluntary instability was not addressed.

Finally, recent literature has focused on the anatomo-pathology of instability including labral tears, capsular lesions and bony deficiencies, which are not addressed by the FEDS system.

4.3 Conclusion

In summary, there is no single classification system that describes all forms of glenohumeral instability currently recognized by orthopaedic surgeons. The FEDS system forms the basis for a new system, but does not include several types of instabilities. A new system, most likely a modification of the FEDS system may prove to be the best system for the classification of shoulder instability.

References

1. Rowe CR (1987) Recurrent transient anterior subluxation of the shoulder. The "dead arm" syndrome. Clin Orthop 233:11–19
2. Rockwood CA (1979) Subluxation of the shoulder: classification diagnosis and treatment. Orthop Trans 4:306
3. Neer CS, Foster CR (1980) Inferior capsular shift for involuntary inferior and multidirectional instability of the shoulder. A preliminary report. J Bone Joint Surg Am 62:897–908
4. McFarland EG, Kim TK, Park HB, Neira CA, Gutierrez MI (2003) The effect of variation in definition on the diagnosis of multidirectional instability of the shoulder. J Bone Joint Surg Am 85:2138–2144
5. Rockwood CA, Thomas SA, Matsen FA (1991) Subluxations and dislocations about the glenohumeral joint. In: Rockwood CA, Green DP, Bucholz RW (eds) Fractures in adults, 3rd edn. JB Lippincott Co, Philadelphia, pp 1021–1079
6. Gerber C, Nyffeler RW (2002) Classification of glenohumeral joint instability. Clin Orthop 400:65–76
7. Jobe FW, Kvitne RS, Giangarra CE (1989) Shoulder pain in the overhand or throwing athlete. The relationship of anterior instability and rotator cuff impingement. Orthop Rev 18:963–975
8. Kuhn JE (2010) A new classification system for shoulder instability. Br J Sports Med 44:341–346
9. Kuhn JE, Helmer TT, Dunn WR, Throckmorton TW (2011) Development and reliability testing of the frequency, etiology, direction, and severity (FEDS) system for classifying glenohumeral instability. J Shoulder Elbow Surg 20:548–556

ISAKOS Consensus Shoulder Instability Classification System

5

Kevin P. Shea

5.1 Background

After reviewing all of the classifications system for shoulder instability in current use, our committee concluded that there is no one single system in current use that could completely classify all shoulder instabilities. As in the case of the rotator cuff classification system, we reached consensus that a new system, based on elements of systems currently in use, was necessary to adequately classify most shoulder instabilities that are reported in the literature. Unlike rotator cuff tears that can be classified visually, instability is primarily a symptom. Thus, any instability classification system should include a classification of symptoms. Five factors were identified as being important in the classification of shoulder instability; 1. Frequency of recurrence, 2. Etiology of instability, 3. Direction of Instability, 4. Severity of instability, and 5. The Anatomic Lesion responsible for the instability. The FEDS system proposed and validated by Kuhn [1, 2] included most of these elements. Our current system is a modification of this system, and thus, a great deal of credit should be given to Dr. Kuhn. The Modified FEDS system is shown in Table 5.1.

We felt that a broader definition of instability was necessary to be more inclusive of most conditions that clinicians currently define as instability. Kuhn defined instability as a feeling of both discomfort and a feeling of looseness, slipping, or shoulder "going out". These elements were included in many other definitions of instability [1, 2]. Using this definition, a shoulder condition that meets both criteria would be called unstable by most shoulder surgeons. However, the definition would specifically exclude the instability seen in the overhead and

K. P. Shea (✉)
University of Connecticut Health Center, Farmington Avenue 263, Farmington, CT 06034-4037, USA
e-mail: shea@uchc.edu

Table 5.1 The modified FEDS classification for shoulder instability

Direction	Etiology	Severity	Frequency	Anatomic lesion[b]
Anterior	Traumatic	Pain[a]	Single episode	Capsule
Posterior	Required reduction	Subluxations	2–5 times	Labrum
Inferior	Never required reduction	Dislocations	>5 times	Bone
	Atraumatic	Locked	Locked	
	Involuntary			
	Positional			
	Habitual			
	Repetitive Microtrauma[a]			

[a] Only applicable to shoulder instability in the overhead and throwing athlete
[b] As determined by either pre-operative imaging studies (CT arthrogram, MRI, etc.) or intra-operative findings. A capsular lesion is diagnosed only if there are no labral avulsions or glenoid bone defects associated with the instability

throwing athlete. This group of patients usually complains of pain in the position of instability but not looseness [3]. They are felt to have "occult instability" or "multidirectional instability" because surgical procedures to reduce shoulder capsular length and volume have been shown to return many of these athletes to their previous level of performance [1, 2]. Thus, these patients have been defined as unstable not because they complain of instability but because an instability operation has produced favorable outcomes in many cases [3, 4]. In the future, a different etiology may be identified as the cause of pain, but we felt that it was necessary to include these patients in our new system. We also included patients with a locked dislocation in the system.

Multidirectional instability and voluntary instability are terms used commonly to classify shoulder instability but the definitions vary according to each study. Neer and Foster [5] were the first to report on Multidirectional Instability, but their case series included patients with a wide variety of conditions and injuries. Like the instability in the overhead athlete, the patients were grouped together because they were treated with the same operation, and in this case, because they all had a positive sulcus sign. Other studies use the term to include patients with some type of instability, but no labral lesion or bone lesion [6]. Thus, we agreed with Kuhn that this term should not be included in any classification because of the lack of specific definition. Instead, the direction of instability should be defined as the direction that produces the most significant symptoms, even if symptoms are produced in more than one direction.

Similarly, Gerber [7] has written that voluntary instability has several definitions including: (a) those who are hyperlax and could voluntarily dislocate their shoulder, but do not complain of any symptoms; (b) those with instability who can dislocate their shoulder but do not do so regularly, and (c) the most concerning group who can voluntarily dislocate their shoulder and do it for secondary gain.

These patients are not differentiated in the FEDS system. However, we felt that each type of instability should be included in order to make the system more comprehensive and inclusive.

The initial reports on shoulder instability by Bankart [8] included the "essential lesion", an avulsion of the anterior inferior labrum, as the anatomic lesion responsible for recurrent instability. Since then, many reports of the treatment of recurrent shoulder instability have included patients without a labral lesion [9, 10]. Recently, there has been a focus on instability secondary to glenoid and humeral bone lesions with or without capsular or labral lesions [11, 12]. Thus, when classifying instability, we felt that it was important to define and differentiate the anatomic lesion felt to be responsible for the instability. The lesion can be defined on x-ray, CT scan, MRI or arthroscopically. If the classification is being used to report the results of a surgical procedure, the anatomic lesion found during surgery should be used. Sub-classifications of the extent of these lesions—percentage of glenoid bone loss—were not included as their significance has not yet been defined [11, 12].

5.2 Modified FEDS System

Regarding the Modified FEDS System, we have maintained all elements of the original FEDS System, modified several elements, and added a classification for anatomic lesions. From left to right the important categories are Direction of instability, Frequency of Instability, Etiology of Instability, Direction of Instability, Severity of Instability, and the Anatomic Lesion.

5.2.1 Direction

The direction of instability is defined as the direction that produces the greatest symptoms. The shoulder is classified as being unstable *Anterior* if there is a history of recurrent anterior dislocations, recurrent subluxations with the arm abducted and externally rotated, or if there is pain or apprehension with the abduction-external rotation maneuver eliminated by a posterior force on the humeral head (i.e. Jobe's relocation sign) or imaging studies (x-ray, CT scan, etc.) document a locked anterior dislocation. Pain alone in the abducted and externally rotated position is only used in the overhead and throwing athlete. Load-shifting maneuvers should not be used alone as it is recognized that many people can have varying amounts of laxity and not have any instability.

The direction is classified as *Posterior* if there is a history of recurrent posterior dislocations, recurrent subluxations produced with forward-flexion, adduction maneuvers, pain in the athlete produced by a posteriorly directed force placed on a forwardly flexed arm, or imaging studies that document a fixed posterior dislocation. Laxity in the posterior direction alone is not diagnostic of posterior instability.

The direction is *Inferior* if there is a (rare) recurrent luxatio erectae, pain or instability primarily with a sulcus test. Inferior laxity with a positive sulcus test is not diagnostic alone; the maneuver must produce the feeling of looseness and pain that is the patient's primary complaint.

We have not included multidirectional instability in the classification for the reasons noted above. Using this system, the shoulder should be examined for instability in all 3 directions with a combination of history and physical examination maneuvers supplemented by imaging studies and the direction that produces the greatest complaint is the primary direction.

Finally, dynamic and static superior translation of the humerus on the glenoid is felt to be primarily related to lesions of the rotator cuff and is not included in this classification.

5.2.2 Etiology

The etiology of the dislocation is defined as *Traumatic*, a single event such as a fall on an outstretched arm resulting in symptoms that become recurrent, *Atraumatic*, if recurrent symptoms of looseness and pain develop without a definite single event, or *Repetitive Microtrauma*—this classification is reserved ONLY for overhead and throwing athletes who develop recurring pain in one position or phase of the throwing cycle. Ordinarily, pain alone, or symptoms not associated with overhead sports are not classified as an instability.

The Traumatic classification was further subclassified into those dislocations that required a reduction after the initial episode and those that were self reduced after the initial episode. There was a felling among the group that there can be differences in the type of instability, with a labral or boney injury occurring frequently with the first type and capsular stretch occurring with the second. There was no actual data to support this separation, only expert opinion.

The Atraumatic classification was also classified according to Gerber's classification of voluntary instability [7]. We defined *Involuntary* as recurrent instability with use and position similar to the recurrent instability described above. *Positional* instability was defined as those patients who could dislocate their shoulder, but the symptoms were painful and they did not do it frequently. Finally, *Habitual* instability was defined as voluntary recurrent instability used purposely for secondary gain.

5.2.3 Severity

We maintained all of Kuhn's recommendations but added the *Pain* with use ONLY for the overhead and throwing athlete and *Locked* for those whose instability has progressed to the point where the shoulder cannot be relocated. *Subluxation* is defined as looseness with a feeling of the shoulder slipping part way out of the joint and quickly relocation. *Dislocation* is defined as the shoulder translating completely out of joint and remaining in that position until some type of reduction maneuver is performed.

5.2.4 Frequency

Using the system, Frequency is defined as a *single event*, i.e. first-time dislocation; *occasional*, 2–5 subluxations/dislocations; *frequent*, more than 5 episodes; and *locked*, meaning that the shoulder is continually dislocated. The division between occasional and frequent is admittedly somewhat arbitrary. However, this is the definition used in the original FEDS system and we did not feel there was any evidence to change it. We have included the locked dislocation for completeness.

5.2.5 Anatomic Lesion

The most significant modification that we made was to include a description of the anatomic lesion felt to be responsible for the instability. All members felt that recurrent instability associated with a labral tear was different in several ways from instability associated without a labral tear. We were not aware of any method to classify labral tears or capsular stretching lesions to further subclassify these anatomic lesions. Humeral avulsions of the glenohumeral ligaments shoulder be included in this category [10]. Boney lesions can vary in size and shape, but these is no consensus on how to subclassify these lesions [11, 12]. Similarly, there is no consensus on the classification of Hill-Sachs lesions [13].

5.3 Using the Modified FEDS System

When using this classification system, we propose that the clinician first identify the direction of instability using history and physical examination. Then using the history, classify the etiology, severity and frequency. For example, a patient could be classified as an anterior traumatic dislocator, who have only one episode. This would correspond to the "first-time dislocator". Then using imaging studies, the clinician might identify a labral tear, a glenoid bone defect, or no anatomic lesion (i.e. capsular lesion). All patients who fit this exact classification could then be pooled from different surgeons, and a larger study could be done with pooled data.

5.4 Future Directions

At this time, we recognize that this system remains unvalidated and that future modifications will likely be necessary. However, we believe that it is the most comprehensive system proposed for the classification of Shoulder Instability to date and suggest that it should be given consideration.

References

1. Kuhn JE (2010) A new classification system for shoulder instability. Br J Sports Med 44:341–346
2. Kuhn JE, Helmer TT, Dunn WR, Throckmorton TW (2011) Development and reliability testing of the frequency, etiology, direction, and severity (FEDS) system for classifying glenohumeral instability. J Shoulder Elbow Surg 20:548–556
3. Jobe FW, Kvitne RS, Giangarra CE (1989) Shoulder pain in the overhead or throwing athlete. The relationship of anterior instability and rotator cuff impingement. Orthop Rev 18:963–975
4. Baker CL 3rd, Mascarenhas R, Kline AJ, Chhabra A, Pombo MW, Bradley JP (2009) Arthroscopic treatment of multidirectional shoulder instability in athletes: a retrospective analysis of 2- to 5-year clinical outcomes. Am J Sports Med 37:1712–1720
5. Neer CS, Foster CR (1980) Inferior capsular shift for involuntary inferior and multidirectional instability of the shoulder joint: a preliminary report. J Bone Joint Surg Am 62:897–908
6. Rook RT, Savoie FH 3rd, Field LD (2001) Arthroscopic treatment of instability attributed to capsular injury or laxity. Clin Orthop 390:52–58
7. Gerber C, Nyffeler RW (2002) Classification of glenohumeral joint instability. Clin Orthop 400:65–76
8. Bankart ASB (1938) The pathology and treatment of recurrent dislocation of the shoulder joint. Br J Surg 26:23–29
9. Jacobson ME, Riggenbach M, Woolridge AR, Bishop JY (2012) Open capsular shift and arthroscopic capsular plication for treatment of multidirectional instability. Arthroscopy 28:1010–1017
10. George MS, Khazzam M, Kuhn JE (2011) Humeral avulsion of glenohumeral ligaments. J Am Acad Orthop Surg 19:127–133
11. Provencher MT, Bhatia S, Ghondadra NS, Grumet RC, Bach BR Jr, Dewing CB, LeClere L, Romeo AA (2010) Recurrent shoulder instability: current concepts for evaluation and management of glenoid bone loss. J Bone Joint Surg Am 92(Suppl 2):133–151
12. Sugaya H, Moriishi J, Kanisawa I, Tsuchiya A (2006) Arthroscopic osseous Bankart repair for chronic recurrent anterior glenohumeral instability. J Bone Joint Surg Am 88(Suppl 1 Pt 2):159–169
13. Provencher MT, Frank RM, Leclere LR, Metzger PD, Ryu JJ, Bernhardson A, Romeo AA (2012) The Hill-Sachs lesion; diagnosis, classification and management. J Am Acad Orthop Surg 20:242–252

Outcomes Scores for Shoulder Instability and Rotator Cuff Disease

6

Guillermo Arce and Kevin P. Shea

6.1 Background

Orthopedic surgeons are encouraged to adopt evidence-based strategies for managing their patients. Levels of evidence have been devised which allow publications to be ranked or given a grade of recommendation. The highest levels are assigned to well-designed randomized, controlled trials and systematic reviews of such trials. Proper studies require good design and the use of validated outcome measure. The use of validated outcome scores allows comparisons to be made between studies. If scores are modified or used on inappropriate groups of patients, such comparisons are flawed.

According to Harvie [4] who reviewed 610 articles relating to surgery on the shoulder, a total of 44 different outcomes scores were encountered. Twenty two were clinician-based (50 %), 21 patient-based (47.7 %) and only one clinician and patient-based (2.3 %). Only 8 (2.7 %) made clear the reasons for the choice of the particular score. Scores may be patient based such as the Oxford Shoulder Score (OSS), clinician-based as the Constant-Murley score (CMS) or a combination of both as in the modified American Shoulder and Elbow Surgeons (ASES). There are condition-specific scores such as the Western Ontario Scores (WOSI and WORC) and non-condition-specific scores such as the Simple Shoulder Test.

G. Arce (✉)
Department of Orthopaedic Surgery, Insituto Argentino de Diagnostico y Tratamiento,
Marcelo T. de Alvear 2400, 1122 Buenos Aires, Argentina
e-mail: guillermorarce@ciudad.com.ar

K. P. Shea
University of Connecticut Health Center, Farmington Avenue 263, Farmington,
CT 06034-4037, USA
e-mail: shea@uchc.edu

In recent years there has been a proliferation of patient-based outcomes scores recognizing the benefits of such scores compared with the clinician-based assessments. The latter are susceptible to bias and error, and may not represent the view of the patient. Patient-based scores are designed for use in clinical trials and are valid for comparing and aggregating cohort studies. Their use will directly improve levels of evidence but many have not been properly tested for validity, repeatability and sensitivity to change.

Despite the trend to move away from the application of clinician-based outcome scores, the magnitude of this shift is highly variable. Over the last decade the use of clinician-based scores has remained high. Investigators planning clinical trials should select modern instruments that have been developed with appropriate patient input for item generation and reduction, and established validity and reliability.

6.2 Published Scores for the Outcome of Shoulder Treatment

Kirkley et al. [6–8] reviewed for the ISAKOS Scientific Committee the most commonly used shoulder scoring systems with their strengths and weaknesses. Other authors described with more details the scores with the main features of each of them.

6.3 The Rating Sheet for Bankart Repair (Rowe)

In 1978, Carter Rowe published a Rating Sheet for evaluating long-term results of the Bankart Repair. There are 4 different versions of the Rowe Score (1978, 1981, 1982 and 1988) [5]. It has 3 different areas: stability, motion and function. The weighting is such that stability accounts 50 points, motion for 20 points and function for 30 points, giving a total possible score of 100 points. It is not clear whether the apprehension is to be measured by asking the patient whether they have apprehension or by examining the patient and doing the apprehension test. The evaluation of motion is not defined as active or passive. This instrument combines 2 items of subjective evaluation with one item of physical examination (Fig. 6.1). This scoring system has not been validated, even for shoulder instability but it is useful for objective instability assessment.

6.4 The UCLA Shoulder Score

University of California at Los Angeles Rating Scale was first published in 1981 by H.C. Amstutz et al. for patients undergoing shoulder arthroplasty for arthritis. The instrument assigns a score to patients based on 5 separate domains: pain,

Assessment	Score
Function	
No limitation in throwing or overhand activities; returned to prior level of competition	50
No limitation in overhand activity; returned to preinjury sport but not at preinjury level	40
No limitation in overhand activity and throwing; did not return to preinjury sport	35
Moderate limitation in overhand activity and throwing; could not return to preinjury sport	20
Marked limitation in throwing; unable to work overhand	0
Pain	
None	10
Moderate	5
Severe	0
Stability	
Negative apprehension with no subluxation	30
Negative apprehension with pain during abduction in external rotation	15
Positive apprehension with positive sense of subluxation	0
Motion	
Full	10
Equal to or less than 25% loss in any plane	5
Greater than 25% loss in any plane	0

Excellent: 90–100 points; good: 70–89 points; fair: 40–69 points; poor: ≤39 points

Fig. 6.1 The modified Rowe score

function, active forward flexion, strength of forward flexion and overall satisfaction. The weighting is such that pain accounts for 10 points, function for 10 points, forward flexion for 5 points, strength for 5 points and overall satisfaction for 5 points, giving a total of 35 points. The items of this instrument were also selected by the authors without direct patient input, similar to the Rowe. Though it has been widely used to report the outcome of rotator cuff surgery, it has not been validated for either shoulder instability or rotator cuff treatment (Please see references [14–16] at the end of the chapter.)

6.5 The Shoulder Pain and Disability Index (SPADI)

Roach et al. published it in 1991. The instrument has 13 items divided into 2 subscales: Pain (5 items) and disability (8 items). The response format selected for the instrument was a 10-cm VAS anchored verbally at each end. The total score for the instrument is determined by averaging the scores for the two domains of pain and disability. Limited validation testing has been described and responsiveness has not been formally tested. No report of the minimally important difference has been provided.

6.6 The American Shoulder and Elbow Surgeons Evaluation Form (ASES)

In 1993, the Society of the American Shoulder and Elbow Surgeons developed a standardized form for the assessment of the shoulder function, including shoulder instability and rotator cuff disease. The instrument consists of a physician assessment section and a patient self-evaluation section [11, 12].

The physician section includes physical examination and documentation of range of motion, strength and instability, and demonstration of specific physical signs. No scores are derived for this section of the instrument.

The patient self-evaluation section has 11 items that can be used to generate the score (Fig. 6.2). There are 2 areas: pain (1 item) and function (10 items). The response to the single pain question is marked on a 10 cm visual analog scale (VAS), which is divided into 1 cm increments and anchored with verbal description at 0 and 10 cm. The 10 items in the function area include activities of daily living as putting a coat, lifting 10 pounds above the shoulder height and throwing a ball overhand. Finally there are two general items: doing usual work and doing usual sport. There are 4 categories for response options from 0 (unable to do) to 3 (not difficult).

The final score is tabulated by multiplying the pain score (maximum 10) by 5 (therefore total possible 50) and the cumulative activity score (maximum 30) by 5/3 (therefore a total possible 50) for a total of 100. The ASES is not disease specific and use in clinical trials may lead to poor responsiveness and validity.

These three instruments Rowe, UCLA and ASES scores have been compared in a group of 52 patients with shoulder instability undergoing surgical stabilization [11]. The 3 scales provided different categorization of patients and correlated poorly with each other.

ASES SCORING SYSTEM

Are you having pain in your shoulder?		YES	NO
Do you have pain in your shoulder at night?		YES	NO
Do you take pain medication (aspirin, Tylenol, Advil, etc…)?		YES	NO
Do you take narcotic pain medication (codeine or stronger)?		YES	NO
How many pills to you take each day (average)?			pills
How bad is your pain today (mark line)? 0 |_____|_____|_____|_____|_____|_____|_____|_____|_____| 10 No pain at all .... Pain as bad as it can be			

Does your shoulder feel unstable (as if is going to dislocate)?		YES	NO
How unstable is your shoulder (mark line)? 0 |_____|_____|_____|_____|_____|_____|_____|_____|_____| 10 Very Stable .... Very Unstable			

Circle the number in the box that indicates your ability to do the following activities:
0 = unable to do; 1 = very difficult to do; 2 = somewhat difficult; 3 = not difficult

Activity	Right Arm	Left Arm
1. Put on a coat	0 1 2 3	0 1 2 3
2. Sleep on your painful or affected side	0 1 2 3	0 1 2 3
3. Wash back or do up bra in back	0 1 2 3	0 1 2 3
4. Manage toileting	0 1 2 3	0 1 2 3
5. Comb hair	0 1 2 3	0 1 2 3
6. Reach a high shelf	0 1 2 3	0 1 2 3
7. Lift 10 lb above the shoulder	0 1 2 3	0 1 2 3
8. Throw a ball overhand	0 1 2 3	0 1 2 3
9. Do usual work – list:	0 1 2 3	0 1 2 3
10. Do usual sport – list:	0 1 2 3	0 1 2 3

Fig. 6.2 The ASES score http://www.orthopaedicscore.com/scorepages/patient_completed_score.html

6.7 The Constant Score

It is the most widely used in Europe for all shoulder conditions [2–13]. It combines physical examination tests with subjective evaluations by the patients. The subjective assessment consists of 35 points and the remaining 65 points are assigned for the physical examination assessment.

The subjective assessment includes a single item for pain (15 points) and 4 items for activities of daily living (work 4, sport 4, sleep 2, and positioning the hand in space 10 points).

The objective assessment includes: range of motion (forward elevation, 10 points; lateral elevation, 10 points; internal rotation, 10 points; external rotation, 10 points) and power (scoring based on the number of pounds of pull the patient can resist in abduction to a maximum of 25 points). The total possible score is therefore 100 points.

The instrument assigned various weights to the items (pain 15 %, function 20 %, range of motion 40 %, strength 15 %). Therefore is weighted heavily on range of motion and strength. This may be useful for discriminating between patients with rotator cuff disease or osteoarthritis but it is not useful for instability.

6.8 The Disabilities of the Arm, Shoulder and Hand (DASH)

This tool was made available by the AAOS. The DASH is a 30 items questionnaire designed to evaluate upper extremity related symptoms and measure functional status at the level of disability. The major criticism of this tool is that the item generation phase did not include interviews with patients with the conditions of interest. It has been well documented that the physicians are poor judges of what is important for the patients.

This instrument is intended for patients with any condition of any joint of the upper extremity. Unfortunately the broader scope of this tool, makes it less attractive for use in a clinical trial for shoulder instability or rotator cuff disease.

6.9 The Shoulder Rating Questionnaire

L'Insalata et al. published it in 1997. The instrument includes 6 separately scored domains: global assessment 15 %, pain 40 %, daily activities 20 %, recreational and athletic 15 %, work 10 %. Therefore the total possible score ranges up to 100. Construct validation through correlations between this instrument and other measures of the shoulder function have not been determined.

6.10 The Simple Shoulder Test

In 1992, Lippitt, Harryman and Matsen reported on the development and testing of the Simple Shoulder Test. It consists of 12 questions with "yes or no" response options. The instrument combines subjective items and items that actually require the patient to perform a physical function. Due to the dichotomous response options, the SST is unlikely to be sensitive to small but clinically important changes in patient function, particularly in shoulder instability.

6.11 The Oxford Shoulder Scores

Dawson et al. first published the Oxford Shoulder Score (OSS) in 1996 to evaluate the outcome of shoulder surgeries other than stabilizations. A second was published in 1999 specifically for shoulder instability surgery. Both scores are 12-item, patient completed surveys requiring the patient to rate his/her answer on a 1–5 scale. The best score is 12 and the worst is 60. Both scoring systems have been shown to be sensitive to changes in patient conditions and should provide reliable and valid information [5, 6].

6.12 The Western Ontario Shoulder Tools

In 1998, Kirkley et al. [6–8] published the first in a series of disease-specific quality of life measure tools for the shoulder, The Western Ontario Shoulder Instability Index (WOSI). The second in the series was published in 2001, The Western Ontario Osteoarthritis of the Shoulder Index (WOOS) and the third instrument, The Western Ontario Rotator Cuff Index (WORC) was published in 2003.

6.13 The Western Ontario Shoulder Instability Index (WOSI)

The item generation was carried out in three steps: review of the literature and existing instruments, interviews with clinician experts and interviews with the patients. The item generation therefore heavily emphasized the patients' opinions as opposed to the expert opinion. The response format selected for the instrument was the 10 cm VAS anchored verbally at each end (Fig. 6.3).

The WOSI has 21 items representing 4 domains. Physical symptoms (10 items); Sport, Recreation and Work (4 items); Lifestyle function (4 items) and Emotional function (3 items). The best score is 0, which signifies that the patient has no decrease in shoulder related quality of life. The worst score is 2100. This signifies that the patient has an extreme decrease in shoulder related quality of life.

The Index correlated predictably with other measures. The WOSI is more responsive (sensitive to change) than other tools for shoulder instability (in order of responsiveness: WOSI, Rowe, DASH, Constant, ASES, UCLA, SF-12 Physical and SF-12 Mental).

It has been shown that clinical examination variables correlate poorly with patients' subjective evaluations of their function. Therefore, clinical examination variables were not included as part of this tool. It is suggested that these data should be collected and reported separately. The WOSI has avoided including any or other caregiver evaluation as part of this tool.

6.14 The Western Ontario Rotator Cuff Score (WORC)

The WORC is a patient completed questionnaire consisting of 21 questions over 5 domains in which the examinee is asked to rate his/her response on a 100-mm line VAS-type response with 0 being the worst and 100 being the best. The 5 domains include: 1. Pain and physical symptoms (6 questions), 2. Sports and recreation (4 questions), 3. Work function (4 questions), 4. Social function (4 questions), and 5. Emotional functions (3 questions). The response to each question is measured in

The Western Ontario Shoulder Instability Index (WOSI)

Clinician's name (or ref) _____   Patient's name (or ref) _____

The following questions concern the symptoms you have experienced due to your shoulder problem. In all cases, please enter the amount of the symptom you have experienced in the last week. (please move the slider on the horizontal line.)

1. How much pain do you experience in your shoulder with overhead activities?	12. How much has your shoulder affected your ability to perform the specific skills required for your sport or work? (If your shoulder affects both sports and work, consider the area that is most affected.)
No pain — Extreme pain	Not affected — Extremely affected
2. How much aching or throbbing do you experience in your shoulder?	13. How much do you feel the need to protect your arm during activities?
No aching/throbbing — Extreme aching/throbbing	Not at all — Extreme
3. How much weakness or lack of strength do you experience in your shoulder?	14. How much difficulty do you experience lifting heavy objects below shoulder level
No weakness — Extreme weakness	No difficulty — Extreme difficulty
4. How much fatigue or lack of stamina do you experience in your shoulder?	15. How much fear do you have of falling on your shoulder?
No fatigue — Extreme fatigue	No fear — Extreme fear
5. How much clicking, cracking or snapping do you experience in your shoulder?	16. How much difficulty do you experience maintaining your desired level of fitness
No clicking — Extreme clicking	No difficulty — Extreme difficulty
6. How much stiffness do you experience in your shoulder?	17. How much difficulty do you have "roughhousing" or "horsing around" with family or friends
No stiffness — Extreme stiffness	No difficulty — Extreme difficulty
7. How much discomfort do you experience in your neck muscles as a result of your shoulder?	18. How much difficulty do you have sleeping because of your shoulder
No discomfort — Extreme discomfort	No difficulty — Extreme difficulty
8. How much feeling of instability or looseness do you experience in your shoulder?	19. How conscious are you of your shoulder
No instability — Extreme instability	Not conscious — Extremely conscious

Fig. 6.3 The WOSI score http://www.orthopaedicscore.com/scorepages/oxford_wosi_score.html

mm and totaled to a raw score. The WORC score is then calculated with the following formula:

$$\frac{2100 - \text{raw score}}{2100 \times 100} = \% \text{ score}$$

Form fields (Fig. 6.3 continued)

9. How much do your compensate for your shoulder with other muscles?

Not at all — Extreme

10. How much loss of range of motion do you have in your shoulder?

No loss — Extreme loss

11. How much has your shoulder limited the amount you can participate in sports or recreational activities?

Not limited — Extremely limited

20. How concerned are you about your shoulder becoming worse

No concern — Extremely concerned

21. How much frustration do you feel because of your shoulder

No frustration — Extremely frustrated

Physical symptoms Score is: 0   0 %
Sports/recreation/work Score is: 0   0 %
Lifestyle Score is: 0   0 %
Emotion Score is: 0   0 %

The WOSI Score is: 0   0 %

Fig. 6.3 (continued)

The WORC has been validated for many languages and in patients with both surgical and non-surgical treatment of rotator cuff tendinitis, tendinosis, partial-thickness tears, and cuff tear arthropathy [11, 17, 18]. The minimal clinically important difference in the WORC is 245.26. In other words, pre- and post-treatment scores must differ by at least 246 points in order to be a clinically significant difference. Measures of statistical significance must also be met.

The WORC is easily administered in an office setting, or through a mailing or e-mail. The scores can easily be entered into a data base for later use (Fig. 6.4).

6.15 Committee Consensus and Recommendations

The Committee considered all of the above scoring systems to measure outcome based on the following criteria. 1. The system should be disease-specific to allow direct comparisons between pre-treatment and post-treatment states, 2. Be primarily patient-completed, or at least to separate physician completed responses and patient completed responses, 3. Include both general health and disease-specific outcome measures, and 4. Be validated for reliability and responsiveness.

6.15.1 Shoulder Instability

It was a consensus recommendation that the WOSI should be used as the primary outcome measure for all investigations on the treatment of shoulder instability. This scoring system is easy to administer either in the office setting or by mail or e-mail. It has been shown to be reliable in documenting differences in patient

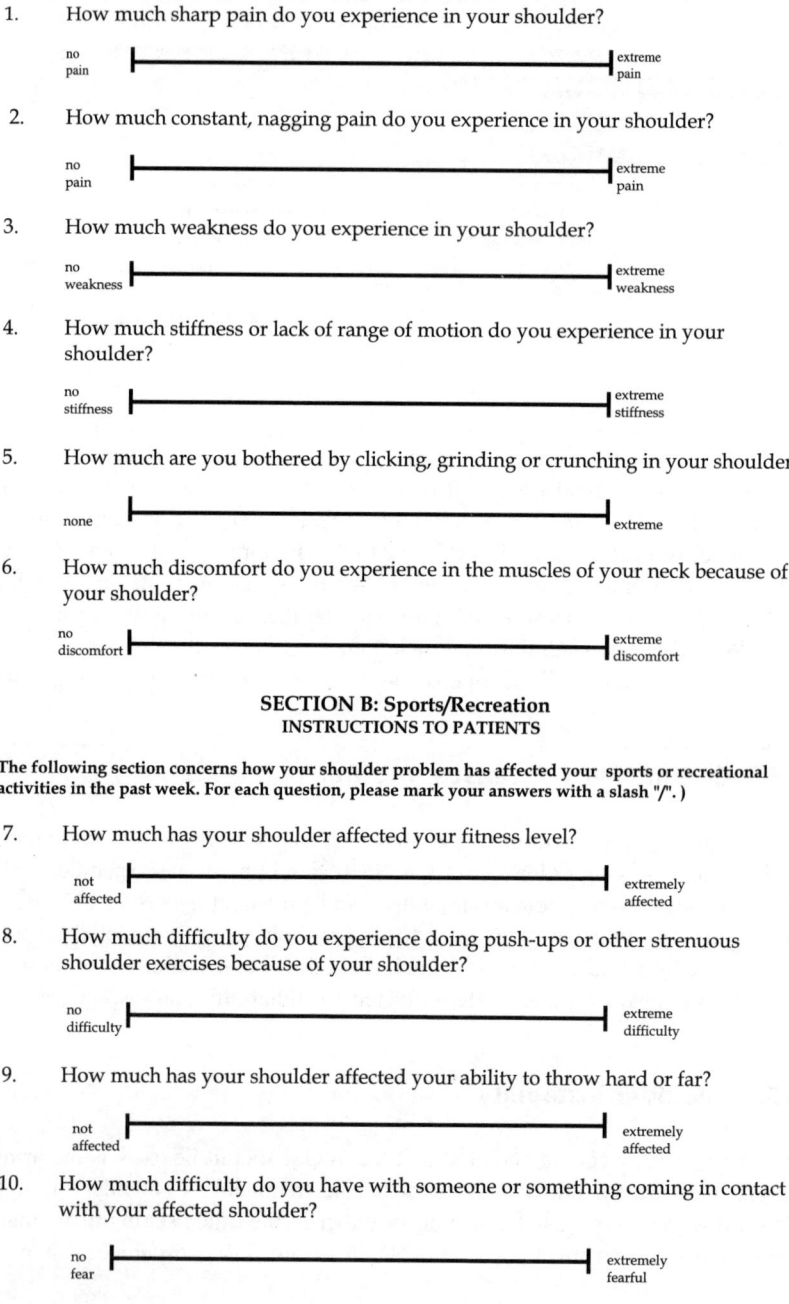

Fig. 6.4 The WORC score

SECTION C: Work
INSTRUCTIONS TO PATIENTS

The following section concerns the amount that your shoulder problem has affected your work around or outside of the home. Please indicate the appropriate amount for the past week with a slash "/".

11. How much difficulty do you experience in daily activities about the house or yard?

   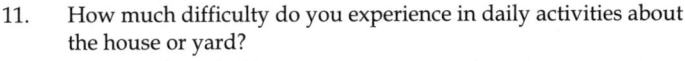
   no difficulty — extreme difficulty

12. How much difficulty do you experience working above your shoulder?

   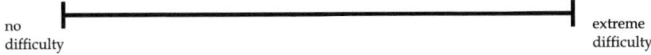
   no difficulty — extreme difficulty

13. How much do you use your uninvolved arm to compensate for your injured one?

   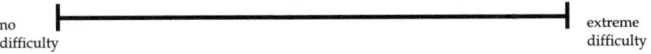
   not at all — constant

14. How much difficulty do you experience lifting heavy objects at or below shoulder level?

   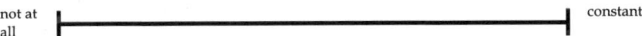
   no difficulty — extreme difficulty

SECTION D: Lifestyle
INSTRUCTIONS TO PATIENTS

The following section concerns the amount that your shoulder problem has affected or changed your lifestyle. Again, please indicate the appropriate amount for the past week with a slash "/".

15. How much difficulty do you have sleeping because of your shoulder?

   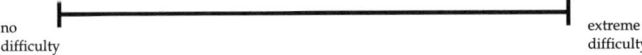
   no difficulty — extreme difficulty

16. How much difficulty have you experienced with styling your hair because of your shoulder?

   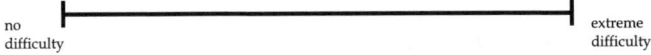
   no difficulty — extreme difficulty

17. How much difficulty do you have "roughhousing or horsing around" with family or friends?

   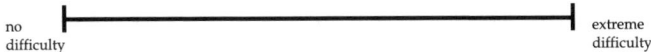
   no difficulty — extreme difficulty

18. How much difficulty do you have dressing or undressing?

   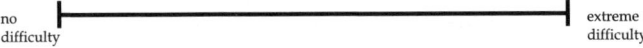
   no difficulty — extreme difficulty

Fig. 6.4 (continued)

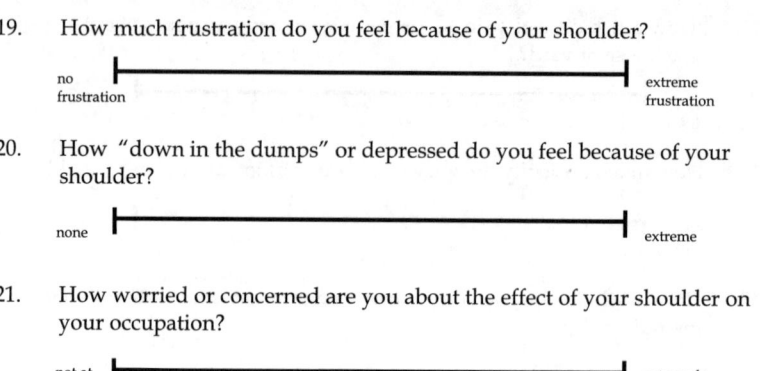

Fig. 6.4 (continued)

condition, includes general health measures, and has been validated for many languages.

Since we continue to value physician completed measures of motion and strength, we made the recommendation that the ASES or Oxford Instability score would be useful as a secondary outcome measure to compliment the WOSI.

6.15.2 Rotator Cuff Disease

The consensus recommendation for measuring the outcome of rotator cuff disease treatment was the WORC using the same criteria as we used for shoulder instability. For a secondary measure of motion or strength, we recommend the use of the Constant Score, as it has been reliably used in many studies of rotator cuff surgery for motion and strength measurements.

6.16 Conclusions and Recommendations

This project was undertaken as a first step of an international organization, ISAKOS, to standardize the outcome reporting of our treatments for patients with shoulder instability and rotator cuff disease. In this way, we hope that we will be able to directly analyze and compare more research and outcome reports and provide even better treatments for our patients. These recommendations are not final and will likely need modification as we use them in our research. However, at this time, it is our consensus recommendation that we should all consider using these scoring systems in our research reporting.

References

1. Balg F, Boileau P (2007) The instability severity index score. A simple pre-operative score to select patients for arthroscopic or open shoulder stabilization. J Bone Joint Surg Br 89-B:1470–1477
2. Gilbart MK, Gerber C (2007) Comparison of the subjective shoulder value and the constant score. J Shoulder Elbow Surg 16:717–721
3. Gerber C (1992) Integrated scoring systems for the functional assessment of the shoulder. In: Matsen FA, Fu FH, Hawkins RJ (eds) The shoulder: a balance of mobility and stability. AAOS, Rosemont, pp 531–550
4. Harvie P, Pollard TCB, Chennagiri RJ, Carrder AJ (2005) The use of outcome scores in surgery of the shoulder. J Bone Joint Surg Br 87-B:151–154
5. Jensen KU, Bongaerts G, Bruhnb R, Schneider S (2009) Not all Rowe scores are the same! Which Rowe score do you use. J Shoulder Elbow Surg 18:511–514
6. Kirkley A, Griffin S, McLintock H (1998) The development and evaluation of a disease-specific quality of life measurement tool for shoulder instability. The Western Ontario Shoulder Instability Index (WOSI). Am J Sports Med 26:764
7. Kirkley A (2002) Scoring systems for the functional assessment of the shoulder. Tech Shoulder Elbow Surg 3(4):220–233
8. Kirkley A, Griffin S, Dainty K (2003) Scoring systems for the functional assessment of the shoulder. Arthroscopy 19(10) (December):1109–1120
9. Kuhn JE (2010) A new classification system for shoulder instability. Br J Sports Med 44:341–346
10. Moser JS, Barker KL, Doll HA, Carr AJ (2008) Comparison of two patient-based outcome measures for shoulder instability after nonoperative treatment. J Shoulder Elbow Surg 17:886–892
11. Rouleau DM, Faber K, MacDermid JC (2010) Systematic review of patient-administered shoulder functional scores on instability. J Shoulder Elbow Surg 19:1121–1128
12. Romeo AA, Bach BR et al (1996) Scoring systems for shoulder conditions. Am J Sports Med 24:472–476
13. Roy JS, MacDermid JC, Woodhouse JL (2010) A systematic review of the psychometric properties of the Constant-Murley score. J Shoulder Elbow Surg 19:157–164
14. Tae SK, MD, Rhee YG, MD, Park TS, Lee KW, Park JY, MD, Choi CH, Koh SH, MD, Oh JH, Kim SY, Shin SJ (2009) The development and validation of an appraisal method for rotator cuff disorders: The Korean Shoulder Scoring System. J Shoulder Elbow Surg 18:689–696
15. Throckmorton TW, Holmes T, Kuhn JE (2009) Intraobserver and interobserver agreement of International Classification of Diseases, Ninth Revision codes in classifying shoulder instability. J Shoulder Elbow Surg 18:199–203
16. Watson L, Story I, Dalziel R, Hoy G, Shimmin A, Woods D (2005) A new clinical outcome measure of glenohumeral joint instability: The MISS questionnaire. J Shoulder Elbow Surg 14:22–30

17. Wessel RN, Lim RN, van Mameren H, de Bie RA (2011) Validation of the Western Ontario Rotator Cuff Index in patients with arthroscopic rotator cuff repair: a study protocol. BMC Musculoskelet Disord 12:64
18. Wessel J, Razmjou H, Mewa Y, Holtby R (2005) The factor validity of the Western Ontario Rotator Cuff Index. BMC Musculoskelet Disord 6:22

Part II
Copenhagen Consensus on Acromio-Clavicular Disorders

Copenhagen Consensus on Acromio-Clavicular Disorders

7

Klaus Bak, Augustus Mazzocca, Knut Beitzel, Eiji Itoi, Emilio Calvo, Guillermo Arce, William B. Kibler and Raffy Mirzayan, and the ISAKOS Upper Extremity Committee

7.1 Introduction

The acromio-clavicular (AC) articulation has received increasing attention the last years. New techniques to re-establish normal function after dislocations have been developed, and arthroscopic techniques for cases of arthritis has been established. The ISAKOS Upper Extremity Committee met in Copenhagen in June 2010 in an attempt to bring conclusions for a consensus on current diagnosis and treatment of

---

ISAKOS Upper Extremity Committee: Vicente Gutierrez, Mauricio Gutierrez, Giovanni di Giacomo, Ettore Taverna, Alex Castagna, Eiji Itoi, Jaap Willems, Steven Cohen, David Lintner, Benno Ejnismann

---

K. Bak (✉)
Parkens Private Hospital, Oestre Alle 42, 3rd, 2100, Copenhagen Oe, Denmark
e-mail: kb@ppho.dk; kb@teres.dk

A. Mazzocca
Department of Orthopaedic Surgery, University of Connecticut Health Center, 263 Farmington Ave MARB 4th Floor, Farmington, CT 06030-4037, USA
e-mail: mazzocca@uchc.edu; Admazzocca@Yahoo.Com

K. Beitzel
University of Connecticut Health Center, 263 Farmington Ave MARB 4th Floor, Farmington, CT 06030-4037, USA
e-mail: beitzelknut@hotmail.com

E. Itoi
Department of Orthopaedic Surgery, Tohoku University School of Medicine, 1-1 Seiryo-Machi, Aoba-ku, Miyagi, Sendai 980-8574, Japan
e-mail: itoi-eiji@med.tohoku.ac.jp

E. Calvo
Shoulder and Elbow Reconstructive Surgery Unit, Department of Orthopedic Surgery, Fundacion Jimenez Diaz, Madrid, Spain
e-mail: ecalvo@fjd.es; emilio.calvo@fmail.com

AC-joint disorders. The aim of this report for the ISAKOS booklet is to sum up the conclusions of the consensus meeting as well as reporting on suggestions from the ISAKOS Terminology Project conducted by the Arthroscopy Committee and the Upper Extremity Committee on a new classification for type III AC dislocations. Part of the consensus was published in the ISAKOS newsletter in 2011, Volume II. The main conclusions of the Consensus meeting in Copenhagen were: that injuries of the AC joint are, a relatively common cause of consultation, easy to diagnose, and easy to classify. Revision options are, however, not easy, and selecting the right patient for surgery may be difficult. Furthermore associated lesions need attention, in particular in patients with grade III or grade V injuries or more. At present the choice of surgical technique and the timing of surgery is still complicated. Regarding outcome of treatment, "failure" needs to be better defined, and there are only few series with an appropriate level of evidence and an adequate number of patients.

7.2 Anatomy and Biomechanics

The AC joint is the only articulation between the clavicle and the scapula. As a result, it bears significant functional importance. The AC ligaments and coracoclavicular (CC) ligaments connect the scapula and the clavicle, and provide stability to the AC joint. The CC ligament is composed of the trapezoid and conoid ligaments: the trapezoid is shorter but thicker than the conoid [1]. The maximum tensile load of the CC ligament is almost twice as large as that of the AC ligament [2]. The stabilizing and controlling effects of the clavicle are passed to the scapula and arm through the AC joint, creating a stable "screw axis", or stable path of coordinated motion of the 2 component bones of the articulation [3, 4]. With an intact and stable AC joint, 3 scapular motions- internal/external rotation, upward/downward rotation, anterior/posterior tilt- and 2 translations- upward/downward, retraction/protraction- occur with normal arm motion. These movements combine with arm movements to place the arm efficiently in optimum positions and motions to transfer the loads and forces to accomplish tasks. In other words, the trapezoid and the conoid ligaments have different functions [5]. Based on this biomechanical

---

G. Arce
Insituto Argentino de Diagnostico y Tratamiento, Buenos Aires, Argentina
e-mail: guillermorarce@ciudad.com.ar; equipo_arce@yahoo.com

W. B. Kibler
Shoulder Center of Kentucky, 240 Market St, Lexington, KY 40507, USA
e-mail: wkibler@aol.com

R. Mirzayan, and the ISAKOS Upper Extremity Committee
Kaiser Permanente 2951 Oakmont View Dr, Glendale, CA 91208, USA
e-mail: lakersdoc@yahoo.com

knowledge, anatomical reconstruction of the CC ligament has been reported [6, 7]. The AC joint is entirely surrounded by the capsule, but the thickness of the capsule is not uniform.

The inferior capsule (mean 1.6 mm) is thinner than the other portions (2.1–2.5 mm) [1]. The AC joint has an intra-articular disc, which usually has a large perforation in the center.

7.3 The Degenerative AC-Joint

The AC-joint is prone to degenerative changes like no other joint in the body starting at an early age, but in the majority of cases it is an asymptomatic finding. MR imaging can be used mainly in the search of possible associated pathology or confirmation of the presence of inferior bone spurs. The disc and the cartilage degeneration is common in the 4th decade or older (8). The prevalence of AC-arthrosis has been reported between 30 and 93 %, more common with increasing age [8–10]. Primary arthrosis of the AC-joint appears more frequent than glenohumeralarthrosis. The prevalence is 8–42 % in grade I and grade II C sprain. An anatomical study showed that the degenerative changes were more commonly observed in the inferior portion of the joint than the superior portion and that the osteophytes were more commonly observed on the acromion, followed by the superior and inferior portions of the clavicle, followed by the anterior and posterior portions of the clavicle (Zuo JL, Itoi E et al.: Anatomic and radiographic changes of the AC jointin an old-age group. In Submission). In a metaanalysis of the outcome of non-operative versus operative treatment of Grade III dislocation, no difference in arthritis was seen [11]. Arthrosis is more common after AC-joint surgery and nailing than after distal clavicle fracture [12].

Open distal clavicle resection (ODCR) consists of debridement of the soft tissue and meniscal remnant, 1 cm resection distal clavicle. The attachment of the capsule varies at different portion of the clavicle and acromion. The objective is to avoid leaving the AC joint unstable, as this may account for some of the failures seen after ODCR. Stine & Vangsness reported in an anatomical study, that the safe amount of bone resection is 2–3 mm on the acromion side and 3–4 mm on the clavicle side [1]. Arthroscopic distal clavicle resection (ADCR) can be performed by the direct or the indirect method. In the direct method a superior anterior and posterior portal is used with a small or regular scope and abrader. The indirect ADCR is done through the subacromial space in conjunction with subacromial decompression. A regular scope and instruments are used to resect 8–10 mms distal clavicle. ADCR aims at preserving the superior and posterior AC ligaments. In a randomized Level II study comparing direct and indirect ADCR, there was a faster return to sports with the direct method and also earlier improvement in ASES and ASSS-scores [13]. In contrast to this Levine et al. [14] found that the direct method was more likely to cause damage to the superior capsular ligaments thereby creating potential distal clavicle instability. In a recent published metaanalysis on open versus arthroscopic distal clavicle resection, Pensak et al. [14] found that the ADCR produces better outcome than the ODCR with success rates of 90 %. Direct ADCR seems to permit a quicker return to athletic activities. A trend toward more "poor" results was seen when distal clavicle excision is performed in patients with post-traumatic AC instability or in Workers' Compensation patients.

In conclusion, the AC-joint is susceptible to degeneration at a very early age. A majority of AC-degenerative findings demonstrated on imaging studies may represent an asymptomatic condition. Symptomatic AC-joint pain has a characteristic location over the top of the shoulder often being tooth-ache like. If non-operative treatment fails, distal clavicle resection preferably should be performed with arthroscopic technique.

7.4 Classification of AC-Joint Dislocation

The most widely used classification is that of Rockwood et al. [15]. It is important to note that this is a purely radiographic classification system (Fig. 7.1). In a type I injury, there is a sprain of the AC ligament only. There is no radiographic abnormality. In type II injury, the AC ligaments and joint capsule are disrupted. The CC ligaments are intact but sprained. There is 50 % vertical subluxation of the distal clavicle. In Type III injury, the AC ligaments and joint capsule, as well as the CC ligaments are disrupted. The deltotrapezial fascia is sprained. There is 100 % superior displacement of the distal clavicle. In Type IV injury, there is posterior subluxation of the clavicle into the trapezius. This is best seen on axillary radiographs. A type V injury is an exaggeration of a type III because of additional complete rupture of the deltotrapezial fascia with 300 % superior displacement of the clavicle. In the rare type VI injury, there is subacromial or subcoracoid displacement of the clavicle [15].

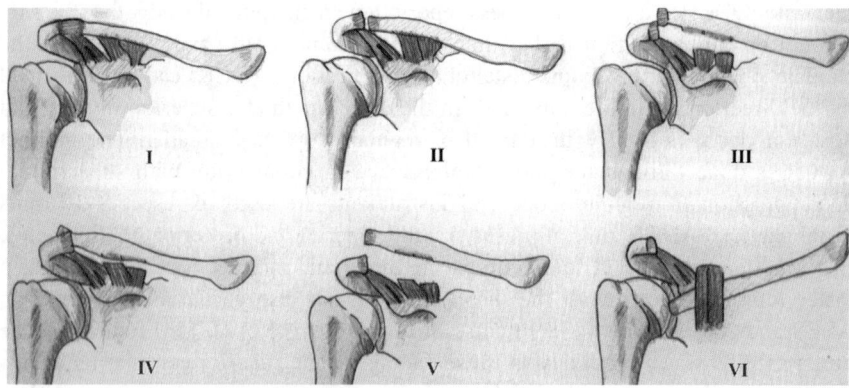

Fig. 7.1 Classification of AC joint injury according to Rockwood's types I–VI

7.5 ISAKOS Terminology Project

Whereas treatment of type I, II, IV, V and VI are generally agreed on, treatment of type III remains controversial. The ISAKOS Terminology project resulted in a new suggestion for the Rockwood classification by further subdividing the type III AC joint injuries into IIIA (stable) and IIIB (unstable) is suggested. The basis for the sub-classification is mainly functional rather than anatomic, but special X-ray views may prove to provide the necessary objective information. The unstable ones will continue to have pain (usually on the anterior acromion, rotator cuff, and medial scapular area), weakness to rotator cuff testing, decreased flexion and abduction range of motion, and demonstrable scapular dyskinesis upon observation. Additional radiographs should be taken to differentiate between stable and unstable type III injuries. We believe that bilateral Zanca views (Fig. 7.2) and a cross-body adduction view (Fig. 7.3) should be added to the routine radiographs [16]. Although there are no published studies, Dr. Basmania has introduced the cross-body adduction radiograph to differentiate between stable and unstable AC joint. If the clavicle overrides the acromion on the cross body adduction AP view, it indicates instability of the CC ligaments in addition to the AC joint disruption corresponding to a type IIIB (Figs. 7.3, 7.4, 7.5 and 7.6).

7.6 Clinical Evaluation and Treatment Algorithm

Clinical evaluation of the scapula should be included in the physical exam of the shoulder in patients with AC separations. It can determine the presence or absence of the alterations in scapular position or motion, collectively called scapular dyskinesis, and can help guide effective treatment of all the functional deficits. A reliable exam can be done within 10 days after the acute injury, when the acute symptoms have decreased. Observation from behind and both arms at the side should evaluate resting scapular position, with visual access to both scapulae. Observation should check for asymmetry of the medial scapular border. This prominence indicates excessive scapular internal rotation and/or anterior tilt, both

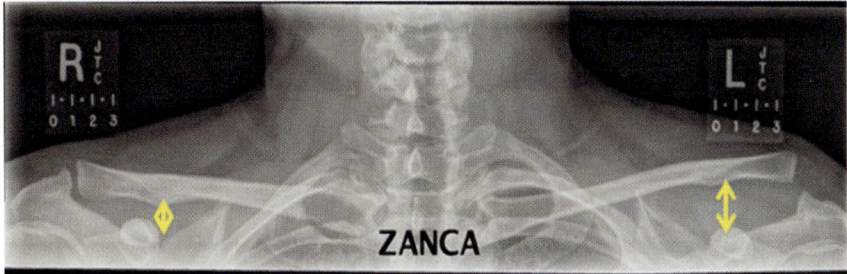

Fig. 7.2 Bilateral Zanca view

Fig. 7.3 Cross body adduction view

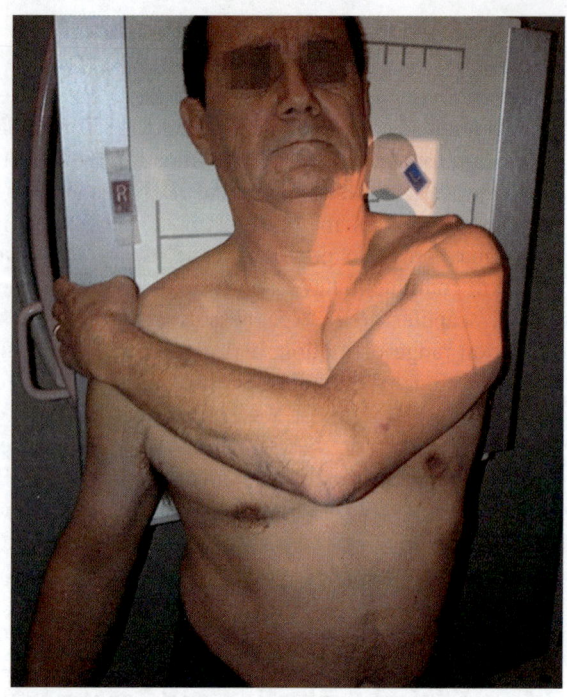

Fig. 7.4 Crossbody adduction view of stable, uninjured side. Clavicle articulates with acromion

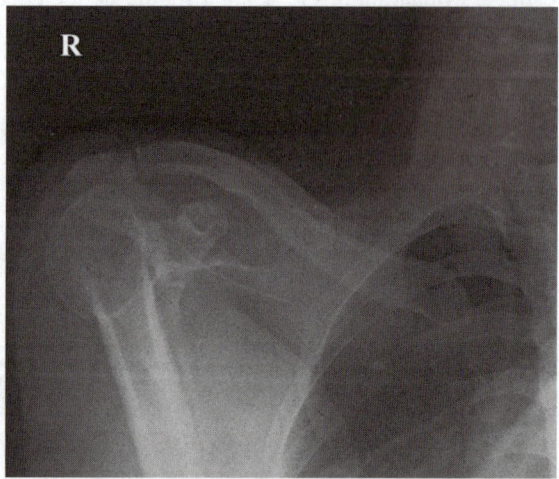

of which can occur when the scapular strut is lost by injury to either the AC ligaments by themselves (type II) or to both AC and CC ligaments (type III and higher).

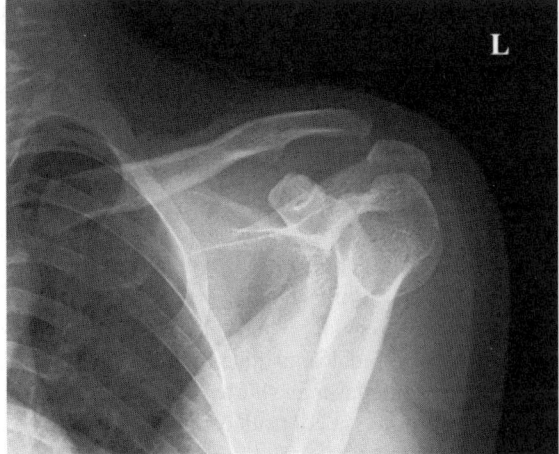

Fig. 7.5 Crossbody adduction view of stable Type III separation. Note that the clavicle does not override the acromion

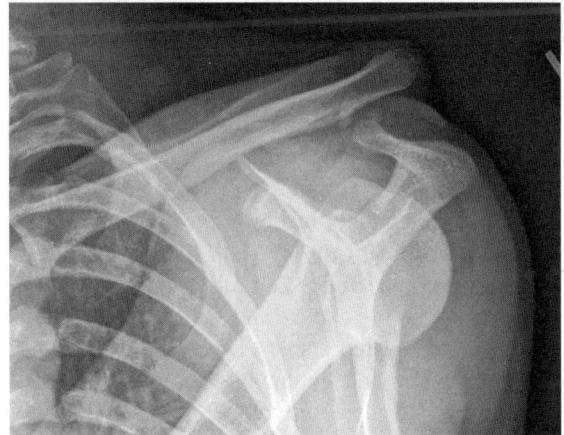

Fig. 7.6 Crossbody view of unstable Type III acromioclavicular joint separation. Clavicle overrides the acromion

The anterior/posterior drawer test as well as the inferior/superior motion test will be positive in AC separations type III and higher, It is occasionally possible to reduce the AC separation by manually reversing the 3rd translation of the scapula, pushing it laterally and then superiorly. If this can be accomplished, the medial scapular border prominence will often be diminished or eliminated, indicating how important the AC joint is to proper scapular position. If this is restored, rotator cuff strength and arm motion in flexion and abduction will also be improved. More often, the AC joint cannot be completely reduced due to interposed tissue. In these cases, scapular corrective manoeuvres such as the scapular assistance (SAT) and scapular retraction tests (SRT) can be used to place the scapula in more normal positions that will improve arm and shoulder function. They will frequently place the scapula in more posterior tilt and external rotation, thereby improving apparent rotator cuff strength, symptoms of external impingement, and improving the ability to achieve shoulder abduction and external rotation. These tests, when positive, indicate the amount of contribution of the scapular dyskinesis to the shoulder problems, and give objective evidence to help guide operative or non-operative treatment decisions.

7.7 Non-operative Treatment

Type I and II injuries are generally treated conservatively with a sling, ice, and a brief period of immobilization, typically lasting 3–7 days. The main goal of this treatment is to eliminate pain and regain range of movement [5]. Attention is drawn towards regaining normal scapula-humeral motion. Additional therapies such as non-steroidal anti-inflammatory drugs as well as intraarticular injection with local anesthetics may shorten the course to a faster recovery, although this has never been proofed in controlled studies. It has to be mentioned, that in some cases of type II dislocation a significant anterior-posterior instability can be demonstrated by the anterior/posterior drawer test, and reconstruction of the AC-ligaments may be indicated, if prior non-surgical treatment failed to remove clinical symptoms.

Type III injuries are often treated non-operatively since comparative studies have reported similar results for conservative and operative treatment, and meta-analyses have failed to find any significant benefit in surgical treatment [17]. Since no clear consensus exists on the management of type III AC joint injuries, the decision is commonly made on a case-by-case basis with an emphasis on initial non-operative treatment [17, 18]. Identifying the subtype of IIIA versus IIIB AC joint separation would be helpful for this purpose. Patients who recover and regain function within 6–8 weeks and whose X-rays show no override on the Basmania view, are considered stable (Type IIIA). Patients presenting a clear override on Basmania view and continuous scapular dyskinesis despite specific functional training are considered unstable (Type IIIB). In light of the controversy and clear lack of evidence supporting acute surgical management of type III AC, we recommend treating all patients (Type IIIA and IIIB) initially with 3–4 weeks of non-operative management. A 4-part physical therapy protocol has been suggested for the non-surgical treatment of grade I, II, and III AC joint injuries in athletes. Phase 1 focus on the elimination of pain and protection of the AC joint through sling immobilization (3–10 days), along with the prevention of muscular atrophy. The authors prefer to start with closed-chain scapular activities that are easily tolerated early in the post-injury period, allowing the patient to work on scapular strength and motion without provoking undesirable increases in symptoms. These exercises unload the weight of the upper extremity, allowing the patient to focus on isolating scapular motion [19]. Phase 2 consists of range of motion exercises to restore full mobility and a gradual progression of strengthening with the addition of isotonic exercise. Phase 3 involves advanced strengthening to enhance the dynamic stability of the AC joint. Phase 4 incorporates sport-specific training to prepare for a full return to prior level of activity. Full rehabilitation should be achieved within 6–12 weeks.

If full function is achieved, but the patient is still in pain, intra-articular injection of local anaesthetic can be used to allow for immediate return to athletics. A patient with an unstable type IIIB AC separation qualifies for surgical reconstruction after a failed short course of non-operative management as defined by persistent symptoms and failure to re-establish normal scapular kinematics [20]. The demands on the shoulder will differ from patient to patient, and these demands should be taken into account during the initial evaluation. Basically return to full motion, no pain and full function with the ability of self protection enables to return to competitive sports [21].

7.8 Surgical Treatment

Operative treatment is generally the accepted method for complete AC joint injuries (types IV, V, and VI) because of the significant morbidity associated with persistently dislocated joints and severe soft tissue disruption [21].

Currently, a wide range of procedures aiming at a permanent reduction of AC joint dislocations exists. However, none of these has been shown to be the "overall gold standard" [21, 22]. Most current techniques focus on reconstruction of the CC ligaments in reference to anatomic studies emphasizing the biomechanical importance of the CC ligaments for vertical stability of repairs of the AC-Joint [21]. Open and arthroscopically assisted procedures are currently known. Of these, anatomic techniques focus on reconstruction of both the conoid and trapezoid ligaments. However, improved horizontal stability may further be facilitated by a reconstruction of the CC ligaments in an early stage after injury with an approach of clavicle and acromion, allowing subsequent healing of the torn AC and CC ligaments and preservation of the clavicle length. Alternatively an additional reconstruction of the AC ligaments could be performed, which is seen advantageous especially in chronic instabilities with decreased healing potential of the AC ligaments. Suture pulley systems can also be combined with free grafts to provide an additional biologic component. Currently, these techniques depend on a minimal tunnel width of 6 mm, which allows for placing only one tunnel in the coracoid in a non-anatomic technique.

The authors intend to demonstrate and discuss only principle surgical techniques. Procedures are separated into open and arthroscopically assisted procedures. Representative for each, an anatomic and a non-anatomic technique are described. General consensus exists that a diagnostic glenohumeral arthroscopy should be performed previous to either arthroscopic or open reconstruction techniques to address possible concomitant intra-articular lesions as described by Tischer et al. [23]. However it has to be regarded, that asymptomatic findings are common.

7.8.1 Open Anatomic

The anatomic coraco-clavicular reconstruction (ACCR) aims to reconstruct simultaneously the CC ligaments (trapezoid and conoid) as well as the AC ligaments for an optimal restoration of biomechanical function (Fig. 7.7) [24]. This anatomic technique restores function of the ligaments with the use of an allogenic or autologous tendon graft (semitendinosus). An accurate anatomic placement of the double band graft at the coracoid represents a key point of this technique. The graft is passed around the coracoid and through two clavicular tunnels, where it is fixed with interference screws. It is vital to place the tunnels at the anatomic insertion area of the trapezoid and conoid ligaments 25 and 45 mm medial to lateral edge of clavicle [25, 26]. The remaining longer limb (exiting the lateral tunnel) is then used to reconstruct the posterior and superior AC ligaments (Fig. 7.8).

7.8.2 Open Non-anatomic

The Weaver Dunn procedure uses the detached coracoacromial (CA) ligament as a retaining structure for the distal clavicle. The modification of this non-anatomic technique involves transfer of the CA ligament to the end of the distal clavicle to restore joint stability with an additional suture construct for increased primary stability [25]. This approach, along with various technical modifications, is still widely utilized to reconstruct the CC ligaments, although not anatomic and considered to be biomechanically inferior compared to the other techniques [21]. Long

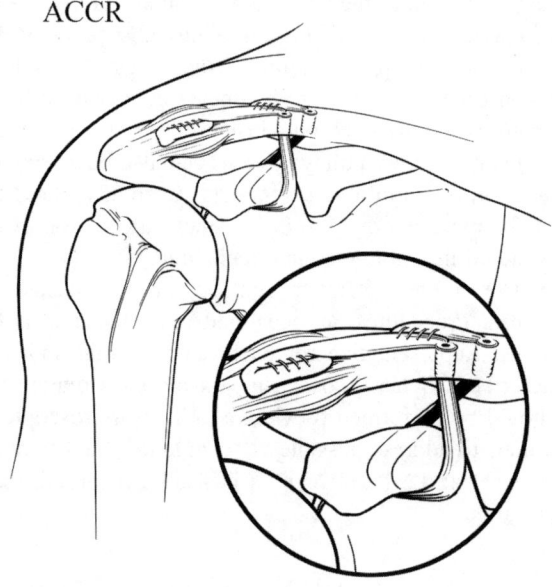

Fig. 7.7 Anatomic coraco-clavicular and acromio-clavicular reconstruction with a tendon graft

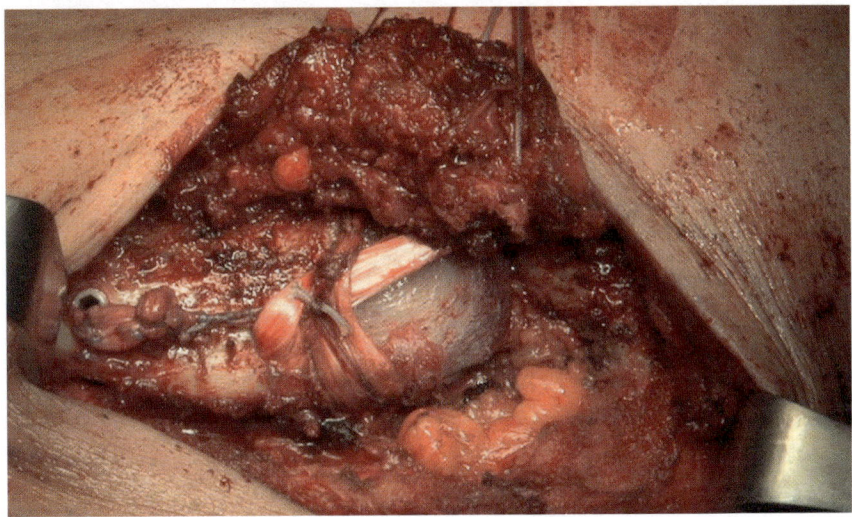

Fig. 7.8 Intraoperative view of the final situs of an anatomic acromicoclavicular reconstruction (ACCR)

term clinical studies need to show if this difference applies to the in vivo situation. A weak point of the ACCR method may be the long distance between the two fixated points of the graft in the clavicle cursing under the coracoid process as compared to the firm and anatomic fixation of the native CA ligament to the coracoid.

7.8.3 Arthroscopically-Assisted Anatomic

For acute injuries, the double cortical button techniques according to the description of Walz et al. can be used (Fig. 7.9) [26]. The basic concept behind this technique is to place one or two cortical button pulley devices through the clavicle and coracoid into an anatomic position corresponding to both the conoid and the trapezoid ligament. Performed in an early stage after the initial injury, this technique is thought to approach the clavicle and the acromion in a physiologic way to promote healing of the torn AC and the CC ligaments [27, 28]. Based on the open anatomic ACCR technique, an arthroscopic modification was developed to pass the tendon graft under the coracoid and through the clavicle tunnels. The potential advantages of the arthroscopically assisted techniques are a more accurate graft placement according to the normal anatomy, resulting in less pain and a more cosmetic result (Fig. 7.10).

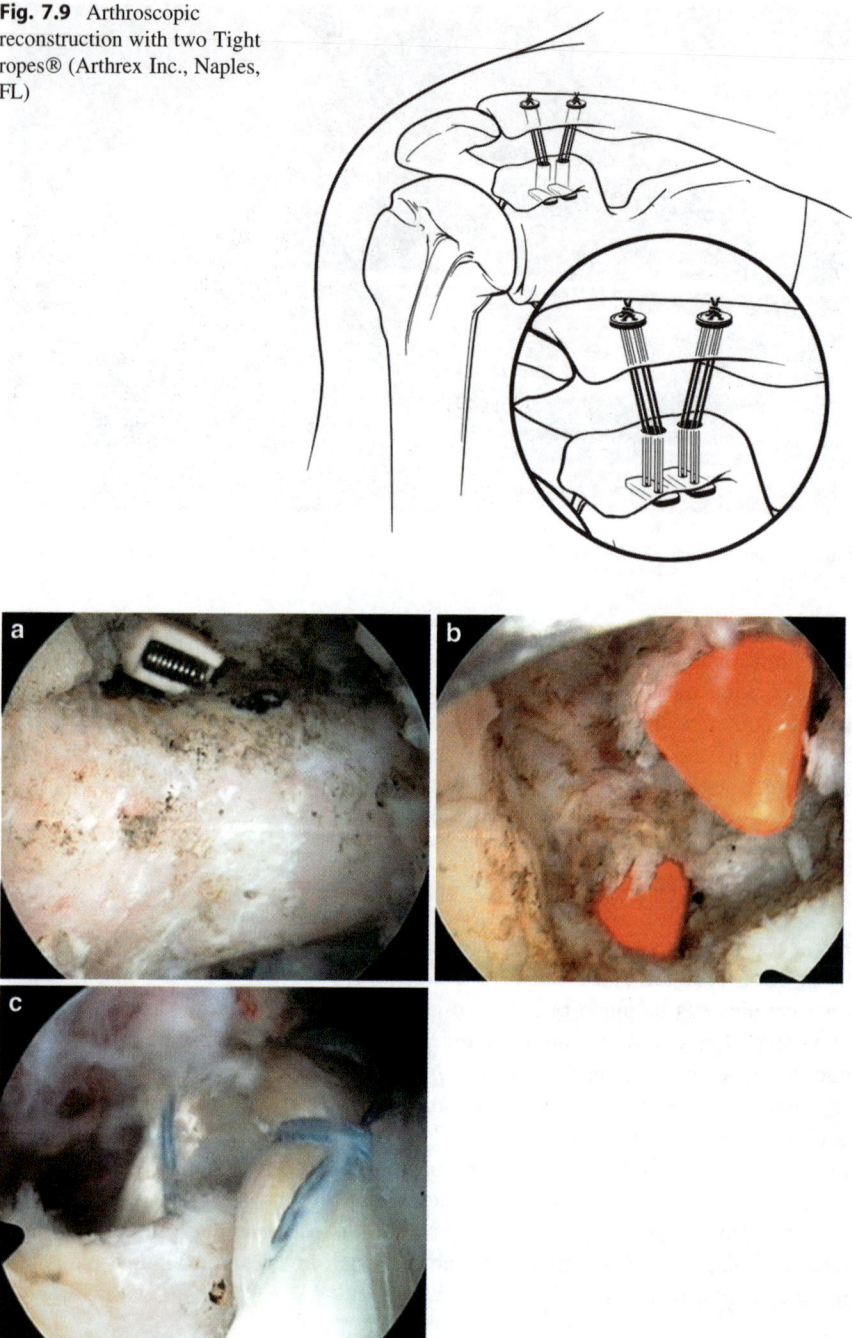

Fig. 7.9 Arthroscopic reconstruction with two Tight ropes® (Arthrex Inc., Naples, FL)

Fig. 7.10 Arthroscopic view of anatomic placement of tendon graft under the coracoid process. **a** preparation of coracoid; **b** clavicular tunnels from below and preparation of graft-passage; **c** final view of both graft limbs passed under the coracoid

Fig. 7.11 Reconstruction with integrated tendon graft (Graft-Rope®, Arthrex Inc., Naples, FL)

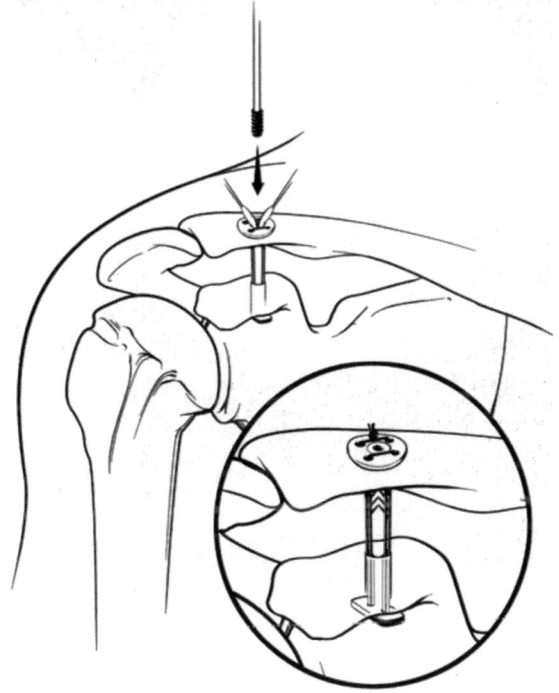

7.8.4 Arthroscopically-Assisted Non-anatomic

Several arthroscopic techniques have been proposed to substitute the damaged CC ligaments, from modifications of the Weaver Dunn procedure to arthroscopic reconstruction of these ligaments with semitendinous augmentation [27, 29]. Single cortical button fixation with semitendinosus augmentation combines a single pulley device with an allogenic or autologous graft (Fig. 7.11 and 7.12). It only reconstructs both CC ligaments as one combined structure and is therefore not regarded as an anatomic procedure. However, it enables to reconstruct the CC ligaments in a feasible one step procedure with a cortical button system for primary stability and additional biology at the same time.

7.8.5 Rehabilitation After Surgery

Directly after surgery for AC joint reconstruction, the patient is placed in a platform brace for the first 4–6 weeks. This provides support and protects the surgical repair against the pull of gravity and excessive loads. The brace may be removed for grooming and supine range of motion exercises only. Following removal of the brace, patients are referred to rehabilitation for active assistive range of motion in all planes. There are no clinical studies to support the degree of immobility in the

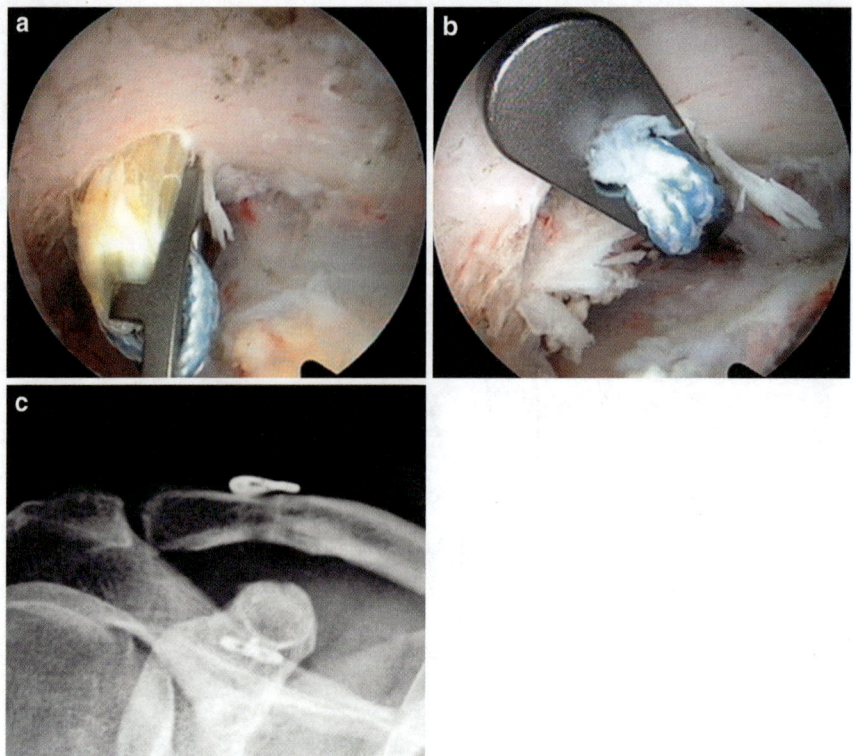

Fig. 7.12 Reconstruction with integrated tendon graft. **a** Arthroscopic view of the graft exit through the coracoid. **b** Single cortical button fixation under the coracoid. **c** Radiographic control showing adequate reduction

weeks after surgery, and in some centers early range of motion, passive and active assisted are encouraged already the day after surgery, but with restrictions in movements that may stress the repair. Motions that may increase stress on the AC- or SC-joint, specifically internal rotation behind the back, cross-body adduction, and forward elevation over 90 degrees, are approached cautiously and within a patient's own pain threshold [19]. The authors prefer to initiate range of motion exercises with limb-supported activities like the table or wall slide. At 12 weeks, if there is a pain free range of motion, strengthening exercises are begun. All isotonic strength activities are withheld for 12 weeks because of concern about the ability of the surgical construct to tolerate a repetitively applied load. However, closed-chain scapular exercises and kinetic chain activities are allowed starting at 8 weeks. From 12 to 18 weeks, exercise is progressed to include isotonic strength activities. Weight training may begin at 3–5 months post-op. Generally it requires 9 months to a year for patients to regain peak strength particularly with pressing activities, or lifting from the floor as in a dead lift.

7.9 Conclusion and Directions for the Future

7.9.1 The Degenerative AC-Joint

Symptomatic AC-joint arthritis is characterised by distinct pain on the joint line and positive cross body test. Non-operative treatment is a success in the majority of patients. Open or arthroscopic resection of the distal clavicle remains a controversy. There may be less morbidity with the arthroscopic approach and faster recovery with the direct arthroscopic procedure. Resection may be limited to less than 10 mm, and resection involving the acromional joint surface spares the AC-ligaments and may prevent instability.

7.9.2 AC-Joint Instability: Clinical Evaluation and Decision Making

The new suggested subdivision of grade III injury by the ISAKOS Terminology Project may improve our possibilities of distinguishing stable and unstable AC-joints. At present this is not possible in the acute stage where all patients are in pain and where provocative tests are inconclusive. We suggest a second evaluation at 3–6 weeks after the injury. The patient must be seen early after the injury by a physiotherapist to regain as much movement and scapular control as possible. If the patient at second evaluation has a continuous functional disability during normal daily life an unchanged abnormal scapular movement, and the Basmania view shows overriding of the clavicle on the acromion, operative treatment is indicated. The authors therefore suggest that the grade 3A and 3B injury are added to a modification of the Rockwood classification.

7.9.3 Directions for the Future

There is a need for clinical controlled studies evaluating the A and B modification of the grade 3 injury and the effect of non-operative treatment addressing scapular dysfunction over regular non-operative treatment. In particular we need to improve our knowledge of the outcome of conservative treatment of type III in overhead athletes from a proper multicenter study.

7.9.4 The Choice of Surgical Method

The choices are listed above. In the acute case there may be a potential for the CC ligaments to heal, and the length of the clavicle can be preserved as well as an attempt to re-establish the joint congruity. In delayed cases it is less probable that the ligaments can heal, and a resection of the distal clavicle end is inevitable. The choice of surgical technique in chronic unstable AC-joints is pointing towards anatomic endoscopic or open reconstruction of the CC and AC-ligaments. In delayed cases, biomechanical studies shows favourable strength of an anatomic reconstruction using a tendon graft over the Weaver-Dunn and modifications. Still clinical controlled studies with long follow-up comparing two methods are lacking in the literature. While there is no doubt that the anatomic reconstruction is biomechanical stronger, the weak point may be when the tendon passes around the coracoid making the distance between the fixation points long and vulnerable to attenuation of the graft. Other future aspects are to enhance ligaments and graft healing with biological augments (PRP or Cell based Therapy).

7.10 Outcome

In order to be able to compare results of treatment of the grade 3 injury, the authors further suggest that a universal standard imaging evaluation to consist of (a) bilateral Zanca view, (b) axillary view, and (c) Basmania view. As no validated disease specific outcome score yet exist, the authors suggest the Western Ontario Shoulder Instability score to be used in conjunction with one other shoulder score. A disease specific AC instability score are under development and can replace these scores when it has been well validated.

References

1. Stine IA, Vangsness CT Jr (2009) Analysis of the capsule and ligament insertions about the acromioclavicular joint: a cadaveric study. Arthroscopy 25(9):968–974
2. Dawson PA, Adamson GJ, Pink MM, Kornswiet M, Lin S, Shankwiler JA, Lee TQ (2009) Relative contribution of acromioclavicular joint capsule and coracoclavicular ligaments to acromioclavicular stability. J Shoulder Elbow Surg 18(2):237–244
3. Ludewig PM, Phadke V, Braman JP, Hassett DR, Cieminski CJ, LaPrade RF (2009) Motion of the shoulder complex during multiplanar humeral elevation. J Bone Joint Surg Am 91(2):378–389
4. Sahara W, Sugamoto K, Murai M, Tanaka H, Yoshikawa H (2006) 3D kinematic analysis of the acromioclavicular joint during arm abduction using vertically open MRI. J Orthop Res 24(9):1823–1831
5. McClure PW, Michener LA, Sennett BJ, Karduna AR (2001) Direct 3-dimensional measurement of scapular kinematics during dynamic movements in vivo. J Shoulder Elbow Surg 10(3):269–277
6. Mazzocca AD, Santangelo SA, Johnson ST, Rios CG, Dumonski ML, Arciero RA (2006) A biomechanical evaluation of an anatomical coracoclavicular ligament reconstruction. Am J Sports Med 34(2):236–246
7. Salzmann GM, Walz L, Buchmann S, Glabgly P, Venjakob A, Imhoff AB Arthroscopically assisted 2-bundle anatomical reduction of acute acromioclavicular joint separations. Am J Sports Med 38(6):1179–1187
8. Bonsell S, Pearsall AWt, Heitman RJ, Helms CA, Major NM, Speer KP (2000) The relationship of age, gender, and degenerative changes observed on radiographs of the shoulder in asymptomatic individuals. J Bone Joint Surg Br 82 8:1135–1139
9. Shubin Stein BE, Ahmad CS, Pfaff CH, Bigliani LU, Levine WN (2006) A comparison of magnetic resonance imaging findings of the acromioclavicular joint in symptomatic versus asymptomatic patients. J Shoulder Elbow Surg 15(1):56–59

10. Stein BE, Wiater JM, Pfaff HC, Bigliani LU, Levine WN (2001) Detection of acromioclavicular joint pathology in asymptomatic shoulders with magnetic resonance imaging. J Shoulder Elbow Surg 10(3):204–208
11. Smith TO, Chester R, Pearse EO, Hing CB (2011) Operative versus non-operative management following Rockwood grade III acromioclavicular separation: a meta-analysis of the current evidence base. J Orthop Traumatol 12(1):19–27
12. Taft TN, Wilson FC, Oglesby JW (1987) Dislocation of the acromioclavicular joint. An end-result study. J Bone Joint Surg Am 69(7):1045–1051
13. Charron KM, Schepsis AA, Voloshin I (2007) Arthroscopic distal clavicle resection in athletes: a prospective comparison of the direct and indirect approach. Am J Sports Med 35(1):53–58
14. Levine WN, Soong M, Ahmad CS, Blaine TA, Bigliani LU (2006) Arthroscopic distal clavicle resection: a comparison of bursal and direct approaches. Arthroscopy 22(5):516–520
15. Rockwood (1984) Injuries to the acromioclavicular joint: subluxa- tions and dislocations about the shoulder. In: Rockwood CA Jr GD, Lippincott JB (eds) Fractures in adults. Philadelphia, pp 860–910
16. Mazzocca AD, Spang JT, Rodriguez RR, Rios CG, Shea KP, Romeo AA, Arciero RA (2008) Biomechanical and radiographic analysis of partial coracoclavicular ligament injuries. Am J Sports Med 36(7):1397–1402
17. Tamaoki MJ, Belloti JC, Lenza M, Matsumoto MH, Gomes Dos Santos JB, Faloppa F (2010) Surgical versus conservative interventions for treating acromioclavicular dislocation of the shoulder in adults. Cochrane Database Syst Rev 8:CD007429
18. Trainer G, Arciero RA, Mazzocca AD (2008) Practical management of grade III acromioclavicular separations. Clin J Sport Med 18(2):162–166
19. Cote MP, Wojcik KE, Gomlinski G, Mazzocca AD (2010) Rehabilitation of acromioclavicular joint separations: operative and nonoperative considerations. Clin Sports Med 29 2:213–228, vii
20. Trainer G, Arciero RA, Mazzocca AD (2008) Practical management of grade III acromioclavicular separations. Clin J Sport Med 18(2):162–166
21. Mazzocca AD, Arciero RA, Bicos J (2007) Evaluation and treatment of acromioclavicular joint injuries. Am J Sports Med 35(2):316–329
22. Geaney LE, Miller MD, Ticker JB, Romeo AA, Guerra JJ, Bollier M, Arciero RA, DeBerardino TM, Mazzocca A (2010) Management of the failed AC joint reconstruction: causation and treatment. Sports Med Arthrosc 18(3):167–172
23. Tischer T, Salzmann GM, El-Azab H, Vogt S, Imhoff AB (2009) Incidence of associated injuries with acute acromioclavicular joint dislocations types III through V. Am J Sports Med 37(1):136–139
24. Carofino BC, Mazzocca AD (2010) The anatomic coracoclavicular ligament reconstruction: surgical technique and indications. J Shoulder Elbow Surg 19(2 Suppl):37–46
25. Rios CG, Arciero RA, Mazzocca AD (2007) Anatomy of the clavicle and coracoid process for reconstruction of the coracoclavicular ligaments. Am J Sports Med 35(5):811–817
26. Salzmann GM, Paul J, Sandmann GH, Imhoff AB, Schottle PB (2008) The coracoidal insertion of the coracoclavicular ligaments: an anatomic study. Am J Sports Med 36(12):2392–2397
27. DeBerardino TM, Pensak MJ, Ferreira J, Mazzocca AD (2010) Arthroscopic stabilization of acromioclavicular joint dislocation using the AC graftrope system. J Shoulder Elbow Surg 19(2 Suppl):47–52
28. Walz L, Salzmann GM, Fabbro T, Eichhorn S, Imhoff AB (2008) The anatomic reconstruction of acromioclavicular joint dislocations using 2 tight rope devices: a biomechanical study. Am J Sports Med 36(12):2398–2406
29. Boileau P, Old J, Gastaud O, Brassart N, Roussanne Y (2010) All-arthroscopic Weaver-Dunn-Chuinard procedure with double-button fixation for chronic acromioclavicular joint dislocation. Arthroscopy 26(2):149–160

Part III
Buenos Aires Consensus on Rotator Cuff Disease: Known Facts and Unresolved Issues

Anatomy (Bone, Tendon, Bursa and Neurovascular Anatomy)

Felix Savoie, Eiji Itoi and Guillermo Arce

8.1 Known Facts

8.1.1 Acromion Shape and the Risk of Rotator Cuff Injury

Three types of acromion shape assessed on scapular Y-view have been reported: Type 1, flat; Type 2, curved; and Type 3, hooked. According to Bigliani et al., 39 % of the general population and 70 % of patients with rotator cuff tears had Type 3 acromion. However, it is not easy to assess the 3-dimensional shape of the acromion using a single plain X-ray. Later, anatomical studies showed that Type 2 was the most common type, with Type 3 being less than 10 % in general population. Also, the contact between the cuff tendon and the undersurface of acromion revealed that shoulders with rotator cuff tears showed wider contact area, which indicated that the acromion shape was more of Type 2 in cuff tear shoulders. Clinically, Gill et al. reported that there was no association between acromial morphology and rotator cuff pathology. Recently, lateral projection of the acromion measured on AP X-ray is reported to be related to the rotator cuff tendon rupture: the cuff tear shoulders showed more laterally projected acromion.

F. Savoie (✉)
Tulane University School of Medicine, 1430 Tulane Avenue, SL32,
New Orleans, LA 70112, USA
e-mail: fsavoie@tulane.edu; ritarichardson08@gmail.com

E. Itoi
Department of Orthopaedic Surgery, Tohoku University School of Medicine,
1-1 Seiryo-Machi, Aoba-ku, Sendai, Miyagi 980-8574, Japan
e-mail: itoi-eiji@med.tohoku.ac.jp

G. Arce
Insituto Argentino de Diagnostico y Tratamiento, Marcelo T. de Alvear 2400, 1122,
Buenos Aires, Argentina
e-mail: guillermorarce@ciudad.com.ar; equipo_arce@yahoo.com

Although the routine use of adjunctive acromioplasty during arthroscopic rotator cuff repair is currently a matter of debate, it appears beneficial in patients with an osteophyte located at the anterior rim of the acromion, in which tendon release from extrinsic impingement is warranted. The lateral acromial edge may also be an important factor in the production of symptoms and should be considered when evaluating the acromion.

In cases of massive irreparable or partially repairable cuff tears, the coracoacromial arc should be preserved even in the presence of a hooked acromion. An acromioplasty in the above mentioned scenario could transform a functional cuff tear into a non-functional one due to anterior–superior humeral head instability.

8.2 Tendon Insertion

Accurate identification of the rotator cuff tear site remains critical for optimal surgical repair. Previous anatomic studies have indicated that the insertion of supraspinatus tendon (SSP) is located on the highest impression of the greater tuberosity, so-called superior facet, while the insertion of the infraspinatus tendon (ISP) is encountered on the posterior portion of the greater tuberosity or middle facet. Nonetheless, recent seminal work by Mochizuki and colleagues, who performed dissection in 103 human cadaveric shoulders, indicates different. In most cases, the ISP footprint was found to cover a large of the portion of the greater tuberosity, while the SSP was attached to only a discrete anterior portion of the greater tuberosity. Thus, the SSP footprint appeared much smaller whereas ISP footprint much wider than previously reported. Of note, in 21 % of cadavers some fibers of the SSP inserted in the lesser tuberosity.

The ISP inserts as two distinct tendons (transverse and oblique). The transverse (superior) tendon blends with the SSP, inserting as a combined tendon on the superior facet of the greater tuberosity. Conversely, the oblique (inferior) tendon inserts lower on the greater tuberosity and in many cases will wrap around the lateral aspect of the greater tuberosity.

Such above-mentioned modifications in tendon footprint anatomy may warrant subsequent changes in current rotator cuff tear classification (i.e. from "U" shape to "L" or "reverse L") and may alter the surgical strategy (i.e., closed with posterior to anterior oblique sutures).

8.2.1 Relationship Between the Vasculature and Rotator Cuff Disease

Blood supply to the rotator cuff is usually provided by the anterior and posterior humeral circumflex arteries and their branches. Likewise, the suprascapular, coracoacromial, suprahumeral and subscapular arteries represent additional sources of blood supply for the rotator cuff. Even though several studies have demonstrated the presence of diminished blood flow at the level of the distal insertion of the SSP, its sole presence does not justify the development of rotator cuff tears.

Moreover, Doppler flow studies (power Doppler, laser Doppler flowmetry and contrast-enhanced ultrasound) have reported diminished blood flow in elderly patients with rotator cuff injury and in cases with impingement; however, an increased flow was found during arm exercise. For decades and supported by cadaveric studies, the mechanism of rotator cuff tears has been considered to be related to inadequate blood supply, especially at the insertion of the SSP. Both, the impact of ischemia in the attritional degeneration of the aging tendon and the whole concept of the "Critical Portion" have been recently challenged by recent Doppler studies showing that the actual area of tendon impingement could be hypervacularized.

8.2.2 The Role of the Subacromial-Subdeltoid Bursa in Rotator Cuff Disease

The medial aspect of the bursa provides blood supply to the rotator cuff tendon that may accelerate tendon healing, and therefore, preservation of this bursa remains essential. Its positive effect along with the presence of anchors holes and the bone marrow derived stem cells enhances the healing scenario for cuff repair. The lateral bursa is often pathologic and a pain generator, which may dictate surgical excision.

In addition, suture configuration should not jeopardize the tendon blood supply.

8.2.3 Bone Quality and Rotator Cuff Repair

Bone density at the level of the greater tuberosity is often weakened with aging, creating a major surgical challenge in patients with rotator cuff tear. In order to achieve adequate screw fixation, the cortical bone in the area of anchor placement should be preserved. The finest bone for anchor placement is normally located on the medial aspect of the insertional footprint, close to the articular cartilage margin. It is advisable to preserve the cortical bone in the area of anchor placement to improve fixation strength. Performing micro-fractures and deep punctures into the marrow should be strongly considered to trigger boost healing factors and stem cells for the repaired tendon.

8.2.4 Suprascapular Nerve and Rotator Cuff Disease

Optimal preservation of the suprascapular nerve remains critical for successful rotator cuff repair. Nerve compression may occur in various regions: anteriorly at the suprascapular notch, at the suprapinatus fossa (by a supraglenoid cyst) or close to the spinoglenoid notch. Recent data supports suprascapular nerve decompression (either anteriorly or posteriorly) during rotator cuff repair. Arthroscopically, this nerve is readily accessible both anteriorly and posteriorly. If the nerve is being compressed by a cyst, the committee recommends cyst resection and debridement prior to superior labrum repair.

The spino-glenoid ligament is inconsistent anatomically, and other nearby structures must be addressed to achieve decompression. Classically, the presence of (a) rapidly progression neurogenic atrophy with positive physical findings (Lafosse test), (b) suprascapular perineural edema and adhesions by non-invasive imaging studies, (c) an abnormal electromyography study and (d) symptomatic relief following selected, guided injection points toward suprascapular nerve compression, strongly supports nerve release along with rotator cuff repair (Fig. 8.1).

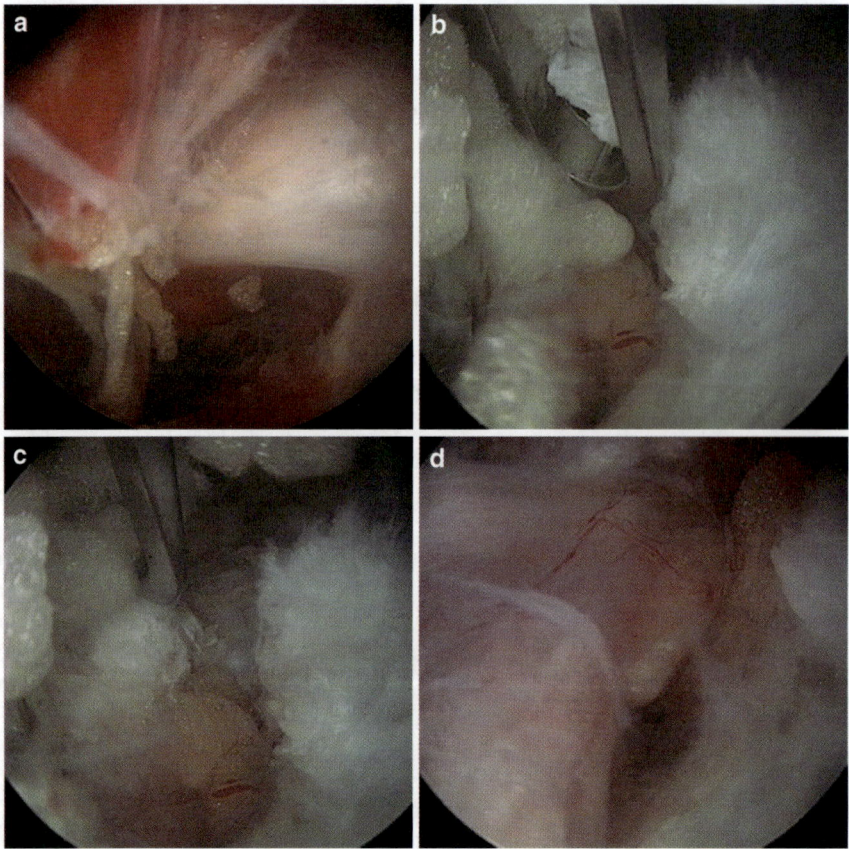

Fig. 8.1 Right Shoulder. Suprascapular nerve release viewed arthroscopically. The transverse ligament (TL) is seen before (**a**) and after transection using an arthroscopic scissor (**b**). The anterior portion of the TL needs further release (**c**). Final result showing optimal suprascapular nerve decompression (**d**)

8.3 Unresolved Issues

Further studies are needed to define whether rotator cuff impingement varies according to acromion type (shapes). The mechanical or biological role of the subacromial decompression needs to be determined with better quality prospective studies. A hooked acromion could be not necessarily the cause of the impingement and rotator cuff tears. The anterior superior instability related to cuff pathology could lead to functional impingement. The potential for reversal of muscle atrophy requires additional research.

The medial bursa provides blood supply to the tendon. However, it is currently unclear if the bursa has to be excised or preserved. Future investigations regarding the appropriate timing for medial bursa reformation after surgical excision as well as the actual role of the bursa with regards to vascular supply to the healing rotator cuff is definitely needed.

The committee agrees that the chronically inflamed bursa has no role other than creating pain. Further researches in vivo are needed to confirm that the bursa reforms after surgical resection and that it has the same positive role as the healthy bursa.

The role of suprascapular nerve release in patients undergoing rotator cuff repair requires further refinement regarding indications and expected results (Please see Refs. [1–25] at the end of the chapter).

References

1. Bigliani LU, Morrison DS, April EW (1986) The morphology of the acromion and its relationship to rotator cuff tears. Orthop Trans 10:228 (abstr)
2. Gallino M, Santamaria E, Doro T (1998) Anthropometry of the scapula: clinical and surgical considerations. J Shoulder Elbow Surg 7(3):284–291
3. Getz JD, Recht MP, Piraino DW, Schils JP, Latimer BM, Jellema LM, Obuchowski NA (1996) Acromial morphology: relation to sex, age, symmetry, and subacromial enthesophytes. Radiology 199(3):737–742
4. Gill TJ, McIrvin E, Kocher MS, Homa K, Mair SD, Hawkins RJ (2002) The relative importance of acromial morphology and age with respect to rotator cuff pathology. J Shoulder Elbow Surg 11(4):327–330
5. Lee SB, Itoi E, O'Driscoll SW, An KN (2001) Contact geometry at the undersurface of the acromion with and without a rotator cuff tear. Arthroscopy 17(4):365–372
6. Nyffeler RW, Werner CM, Sukthankar A, Schmid MR, Gerber C (2006) Association of a large lateral extension of the acromion with rotator cuff tears. J Bone Joint Surg Am 88(4):800–805
7. Mochizuki T, Sugaya H, Uomizu M, Maeda K, Matsuki K, Sekiya I, Muneta T, Akita K (2009) Humeral insertion of the supraspinatus and infraspinatus. New anatomical findings regarding the footprint of the rotator cuff. Surgical technique. J Bone Joint Surg Am 91(Suppl 2 Pt 1):1–7
8. Rothman RH, Parke WW (1965) The vascular anatomy of the rotator cuff. Clin Orthop Relat Res 41:176–186
9. Codman EA (1934) The shoulder. Thomas Todd, Boston

10. Levy O, Relwani J, Zaman T, Even T, Venkateswaran B, Copeland S (2008) Measurement of blood flow in the rotator cuff using laser Doppler flowmetry. J Bone Joint Surg Br 90(7):893–898
11. Adler RS, Fealy S, Rudzki JR, Kadrmas W, Verma NN, Pearle A, Lyman S, Warren RF (2008) Rotator cuff in asymptomatic volunteers: contrast-enhanced US depiction of intratendinous and peritendinous vascularity. Radiology 248(3):954–961
12. Funakoshi T, Iwasaki N, Kamishima T, Nishida M, Ito Y, Kondo M, Minami A (2010) In vivo visualization of vascular patterns of rotator cuff tears using contrast-enhanced ultrasound. Am J Sports Med 38(12):2464–2471
13. Uhthoff HK, Sarkar K (1991) Surgical repair of rotator cuff ruptures. The importance of the subacromial bursa. J Bone Joint Surg Br 73(3):399–401
14. Lewis JS, Raza SA, Pilcher J, Heron C, Poloniecki JD (2009) The prevalence of neovascularity in patients clinically diagnosed with rotator cuff tendinopathy. BMC Musculoskelet Disord 21(10):163
15. Meyer DC, Fucentese SF, Koller B, Gerber C (2004) Association of osteopenia of the humeral head with full-thickness rotator cuff tears. J Shoulder Elbow Surg 13(3):333–337
16. Boykin RE, Friedman DJ, Higgins LD, Warner JJP (2010) Suprascapular neuropathy. J Bone Joint Surg Am 92:2348–2364
17. Bhatia DN, de Beer JF, van Rooyen KS, du Toit DF (2006) Arthroscopic suprascapular nerve decompression at the suprascapular notch. Arthroscopy 22(9):1009–1013
18. Brown KE, Sticker L (2011) Shoulder pain and dysfunction secondary to neural injury. Int J Sports Phys Ther 6(3):224–233
19. Costouros JG, Porramatikul MP, Lie DT, Warner JJP (2007) Reversal of suprascapular neuropathy following arthroscopic repair of massive supraspinatus and infraspinatus rotator cuff tears. Arthroscopy 23(11):1152–1161
20. Cummins CA, Messer TM, Nuber G (2000) Current concepts review. Suprascapular nerve entrapment. J Bone Joint Surg Am 82(A3):415–424
21. Ghodadra AN, Nho SJ, Verma MM, Reiff S, Piasecki DP, Provencher MT, Romeo AA (2009) Arthroscopic decompression of the suprascapular nerve at the spinoglenoid notch and suprascapular notch through the subacromial space. Arthroscopy 25(4):439–445
22. Lafosse L, Tomasi A, Corbett S, Baier G, Willems K, Gobezie R (2007) Arthroscopic release of suprascapular nerve entrapment at the suprascapular notch: technique and preliminary results. Arthroscopy 23(1):34–42
23. Lafosse L, Piper K, Lanz U (2011) Arthroscopic suprascapular nerve release: indications and technique. J Shoulder Elbow Surg 20:S9–S13
24. Plancher KD, Luke TA, Peterson RK, Yacoubian SV (2007) Posterior shoulder pain: a dynamic study of the spinoglenoid ligament and treatment with arthroscopic release of the scapular tunnel. Arthroscopy 23(9):991–998
25. Romeo AA, Ghodadra NS, Salata MJ, Provencher MT (2010) Arthroscopic suprascapular nerve decompression: indications and surgical technique. J Shoulder Elbow Surg 19:118–123

Biomechanics

Ben Kibler and Giovanni Di Giacomo

9.1 Known Facts

The shoulder represents a closed chain system where the humeral head is positioned for function by a closed chain formed by the thorax (kinetic chain), scapula, and clavicle. The purpose of a closed chain kinetic system is to provide stability (ball and socket kinematics) with maximal motion (mobility). Changes in elements of the aforementioned system will influence the kinematic and dynamic behaviour of the other elements within the system. Any rotator cuff activation will require some response (stabilization, change) within the system and may affect rotator cuff activation, compression, tension or motion. Kinetic chain activity affects the capability of the rotator cuff to develop strength and act as a compressor cuff to produce effective force couples and to be active throughout the entire range of shoulder motion. The shoulder works biomechanically as a funnel to regulate and transfer forces from the engine (trunk and core) to the delivery mechanism (hand). Except for extremes of shoulder motion, the rotator cuff musculature provides a very large proportion of the dynamic glenohumeral stability.

The scapula, on the other hand, plays a critical role in glenohumeral function by offering a stable base for muscle activation and load transfer within the closed kinetic chain. Abnormalities in normal scapular position or kinematics can affect rotator cuff function.

B. Kibler (✉)
Shoulder Center of Kentucky, 240 Market St, Lexington, KY 40507, USA
e-mail: wkibler@aol.com

G. Di Giacomo
Concordia Hospital for Special Surgery, Via delle Sette Chiese, 90, 145 Rom, Italy
e-mail: concordia@iol.it

Hence, scapular position and motion have major effects on compression and tensile strain of the rotator cuff, biceps, and superior labrum. Alterations in scapular motion and position are frequent in patients with impingement and rotator cuff injury, resulting into less upward rotation, increased anterior tilt, and less external rotation. In addition, increased upper trapezius activation is normally encountered in an effort to elevate the entire shoulder system and allow arm motion and shoulder strength.

Functional scores in patients with rotator cuff tears are strongly dependant on scapular function. Maximal demonstrated rotator cuff strength capability is related to a stabilized scapular position.

Internal impingement, partial undersurface rotator cuff tears, superior labral tears, glenohumeral internal rotation deficit (GIRD) and total range of motion deficit (TROMD), are all frequently related in etiology and clinical presentation. In overhead demand patients, superior labral tear from anterior to posterior (SLAP), GIRD, TROMD, and anterior laxity appear to be associated with partial thickness undersurface rotator cuff tears.

9.2 Unresolved Issues

How the altered proximal motions and force development relate to rotator cuff injury causation, cuff tear progression, and decisions for treatment.

It is unclear whether altered proximal activations and motions are always associated with rotator cuff injury, if they are; it is unknown whether they are the cause or the result of rotator cuff injury.

The most effective methods of clinically evaluating the altered kinetic chain and scapular factors.

The exact role of internal impingement in partial rotator cuff injuries.

The effect of using kinetic chain conditioning methods in prevention of rotator cuff injuries in susceptible populations.

9.3 Suggestions for Future Directions of Research and Education

Knowledge that the rotator cuff injuries do not occur in isolation, and are not the only factors relating to the patient complaints, but are a part of the entire patient dysfunction. Clinical methods of evaluation of the kinetic chain and scapula.

Effective rehabilitation methods utilizing the kinetic chain based rehabilitation program (Please see Refs. [1–17] at the end of the chapter).

References

1. Burkhart SS (1994) Reconciling the paradox of rotator cuff repair versus debridement a unified biomechanical rationale for the treatment of rotator cuff tears. Arthroscopy 10:4–19
2. Burkhart SS (1992) Fluoroscopic comparison of kinematic patterns in massive rotator cuff tears. Clin Orthop Relat Res 284:144–152
3. Di Giacomo G, Pouliart N, Costantini A, De Vita A (2008) Atlas of functional shoulder anatomy. Springer, New York
4. Gerber G, Fuchs B, Hodler J (2000) The result of repair of massive tears of the rotator cuff. J Bone Joint Surg Am 82:505–515
5. Kibler WB (1995) Biomechanical analysis of the shoulder during tennis activities. Clin Sports Med 14:79–85
6. Kibler WB (2000) Evaluation and diagnosis of scapulothoracic problems in the athlete. Sports Med Arthrosc Rev 8:192–202
7. Kibler WB, Dome DC (2012) Internal impingement: concurrent superior labral and rotator cuff injuries. Sports Med Arthrosc Rev 20(1):30–33
8. Kibler WB (2012) The scapula in rotator cuff disease. Med Sport Sci 57:27–40
9. Kibler WB, Ludewig PM, McClure PW, Uhl TL, Sciascia AD (2009) Scapula summit 2009. J Orthop Sports Phys Ther 39(11):A1–A13
10. Kibler WB (2001) Livingston BP Closed-chain rehabilitation for upper and lower extremities. J Am Acad Orthop Surg 9:412–421
11. Lephart SM, Warner JP, Borsa PA, Fu FH (1994) Proprioception of the shoulder joint in healthy, unstable, and surgically repaired shoulders. J Shoulder Elbow Surg 3:371–380
12. Ludewig PM, Phadke V, Braman JP, Hassett DR, Cicminski CJ, LaPrade RF (2009) Motion of the shoulder complex during multiplanar humeral elevation. J Bone Joint Surg (Am) 91A(2):378–389
13. Ludewig PM, Reynolds JF (2009) The association of scapular kinematics and glenohumeral joint pathologies. J Orthop Sports Phys Ther 39(2):90–104
14. Mell AG, LaScalza S, Guffey P, Carpenter JE, Hughes RE (2005) Effect of rotator cuff pathology on shoulder rhythm. J Shoulder Elbow Surg 14:S58–S64
15. Vangsness CT, Ennis M, Taylor JG, Atkinson R (1995) Neural Anatomy of the glenohumeral ligaments, labrum and subacromial bursa. Arthroscopy 11:180–184
16. Veeger HEJ, van der Helm FCT (2007) Shoulder function: the perfect compromise between mobility and stability. J Biomech 40:2119–2129
17. Winter DA (1990) Biomechanics and motor control of human movement, 2nd edn. Wiley Interscience, New York, pp 191–212

Tendinosis, Impingement and Ruptures

10

Klaus Bak, Eiji Itoi, Augustus Mazzocca and Tom Ludvigsen

10.1 Diagnosis of the Symptomatic Rotator Cuff Tear

10.1.1 Known Facts

Data collection regarding the mechanism of injury, degree and type of pain, clinical dysfunction as well as patient's demands contributes to an accurate diagnosis of rotator cuff tear and can guide future treatment. The clinical examination is at least equal, if not more, accurate than any technology.

Up until now, no single test has provided high accuracy; usually they have either high sensitivity or specificity but not both. For example, in the setting of an acute rotator cuff tear, the presence of impingement signs is very sensitive that lacks specificity.

K. Bak (✉)
Parkens Private Hospital, Oestre Alle 42, 3rd, 2100, Copenhagen Oe, Denmark
e-mail: kb@ppho.dk; kb@teres.dk

E. Itoi
Department of Orthopaedic Surgery, Tohoku University School of Medicine,
1-1 Seiryo-Machi, Aoba-ku, Sendai, Miyagi 980-8574, Japan
e-mail: itoi-eiji@med.tohoku.ac.jp

A. Mazzocca
Department of Orthopaedic Surgery, University Of Connecticut Health Center, 263 Farmington Ave MARB 4th Floor, Farmington, CT 06030-4037, USA
e-mail: mazzocca@uchc.edu; Admazzocca@Yahoo.Com

T. Ludvigsen
Oslo University Hospital, Kirkeveien 166, 454, Oslo, Norway
e-mail: tomcl@getmail.no; tolu@uus.no

Conversely, cuff specific tests such as the drop arm test, the External Rotational Lag sign (ERLS), the Whipple's test (complete SS tear) and the Internal Rotational Lag sign (IRLS for subscapularis) are quite specific but not sensitive.

The subacromial injection of lidocaine enables assessment of passive range of motion and cuff strength. Of note, its use improves specificity of cuff specific tests (>90 %) while reducing their sensitivity. For the impingement signs, the same pattern is seen, though the specificity is reduced [1].

Scapular dyskinesia is a commonly encountered sign in patients with symptomatic tears though not very specific.

A meta-analysis of various cohort studies found the overall sensitivity and specificity of a clinical exam to rule out a full-thickness rotator cuff tear to be 90 %. Thus, combined test (2–4) improves diagnostic accuracy reaching magnetic resonance imaging (MRI) levels.

Further confirmation of rotator cuff tear requires non-invasive imaging (i.e. X-ray followed by ultrasound or MRI).

10.1.2 Unresolved Issues

The actual cause of symptomatology after rotator cuff tear remains unclear. We do not know what is responsible for the symptoms.

10.1.3 Research and Education

Develop a simple and reproducible set of diagnostic tests and questions to evaluate the patient with rotator cuff symptoms that can be repeated post treatment to evaluate the effectiveness of said treatment. Such tests would require further validation.

10.2 Acromioplasty 2012: Is There an Indication?

10.2.1 Known Facts

Non-operative management of impingement is effective in the vast majority of cases. Surgical indications for isolated acromioplasty have been decreasing due to refinement in clinical examination and non-invasive imaging studies. Primary indication for acromioplasty is the presence of lateral shoulder pain aggravated at night, positive impingement signs, a painful arc with no improvement on scapular assistance test (SAT) and scapular retraction test (SRT). This procedure is best indicated in patients not benefiting from a 3-month rehabilitation program.

There is no statistical difference in rotator cuff repair (RCR) healing rates with and without acromioplasty [2, 3], and there is evidence to suggest no reduction in long term re-tear rate when acromioplasty is performed at the index repair [4]. There may be some role for evaluation and decompression of the lateral acromion, as shown by Gerber in rotator cuff tears.

10.2.2 Unresolved Issues

The mechanism by which the sub-acromial decompression works.

It has never been proven that surgery for isolated impingement is better than rehabilitative treatment.

10.2.3 Future Directions for Research

Direct comparison studies of isolated acromioplasty versus current rehabilitation program for patients with classical impingement syndrome are needed.

10.3 Coracoid Impingement

10.3.1 Known Facts

Primary coracoid impingement occurs from spurs, subscapularis tendon calcification and is due to a decrease of the coracohumeral distance. The most reliable clinical test is the modified Hawkins-Kennedy impingement sign, in which the arm is positioned in abduction of 45–60°, forward flexion and internal rotation with a slight anterior subluxation force. The occurrence of symptoms, grinding and pain are indicative of coracoid impingement. In addition, pain at the coracoid tip is a common finding in this patient population.

Diagnostic imaging has been recommended. The role of the measuring the "coracoid index" (coracohumeral distance) is not well defined. In most cases a simple axillary radiograph is an accurate as more advanced imaging in evaluating the posterior projection of the coracoid. Patients with coracoid impingement may have narrowed coracohumeral intervals. Friedman et al. [5] evaluated the coracohumeral interval on dynamic MRI. Asymptomatic patients were found to have an average coracohumeral interval of 11 mm, whereas symptomatic patients had a mean coracohumeral interval of 5.5 mm. However, the exact number that defines impingement has not yet been defined.

Non-surgical management for suspected coracoid impingement is currently recommended for 3–6 months, in which rehabilitation exercises are focused on improving posture and scapular retraction to open the sub-coracoid interval.

Coracoid decompression is indicated in patients with positive impingement findings, positive injection sign and a failure of conservative measures. Surgery is performed arthroscopically, with removal of the posterior part of the tip of the coracoid that projects beyond the origin of the conjoined tendon.

10.3.2 Unresolved Issues

The normal coracoid anatomic variants are yet to be defined.

It is unknown how to perform a precise impingement diagnosis.

The exact amount of bone removal required during coracoid decompression is still a matter of debate.

No one has looked at outcomes of nonoperative physical therapy treatment.

The best surgical technique has yet to be defined in terms of arthroscopic versus open.

The prevalence and incidence of this condition has yet to be defined.

10.4 How and Why the Tendon Fails?

10.4.1 Known Facts

The biopsy specimens of retrieved tendon from rotator cuff tears have demonstrated disorganized collagen, scar tissue and minimal attempts of a healing process.

According to Tuoheti et al. [6], age related tendinosis plus apoptosis phenomenon leads to tendon failure. Apoptosis is a form of cell death in which a programmed sequence of events leads to the elimination of cells. Apoptosis plays a crucial role in developing and maintaining the health of the body by eliminating old cells, unnecessary cells, and unhealthy cells. The human body replaces perhaps one million cells per second. Too little or too much apoptosis can play a role in many diseases.

10.4.2 Unresolved Issues

The correlation between subacromial impingement and tendon failure needs further investigation. So far it has been shown that the apoptotic index increase with impingement and rotator cuff tears.

10.5 Tear Retraction Patterns

10.5.1 Known Facts

In most cases the tendon retracts along the line of pull of the muscle fibers.

The rotator cuff tendon degenerates and weakens with age and demonstrates a specific area of high stress concentration at the articular side of the supraspinatus close to its most anterior attachment site near the biceps tendon.

Several factors have been associated with tear development (i.e., tendinosis, keel type acromion and hardening of the coraco-acromial ligament). Both mechanisms, tendinosis and friction, may cause in concert a tendon tear.

The presence of a more lateral and anterior acromion overhang leads to an increased supraspinatus tendon workload and friction with the acromion, and this is believed to be associated with the development of tendon tear.

The occurrence and the depth of the bursal-side tear appear to be related to the coraco-acromial arch.

Tear propagation runs anteriorly and posteriorly at a rate of 5 mm per year. Smoking and heavy labor amplify tear propagation.

10.6 Asymptomatic Tears

10.6.1 Known Facts

Size and location are the most important factors in consideration of the management of asymptomatic tears. Baseline size and location of asymptomatic rotator cuff tears may predict symptomatic progression. Most asymptomatic rotator cuff tears responded to non-operative protocols and remained asymptomatic at 2 years.

According to Yamaguchi, when an asymptomatic tear becomes symptomatic, we have to beware about an increase of the tear size.

10.7 Unresolved Issues

What triggers symptoms in patients with rotator cuff tears? Soifer et al. [7] suggested that free nerve endings in rotator cuff tendon, biceps tendon and biceps sheath, and the subacromial bursa may relay nociceptive information; however, the original event that triggers this relay remains unclear.

Is there a relationship between tear pattern and shoulder pain?

Is the pain provoked by the anatomic lesion or by the functional impairment of the shoulder?

What are the long term consequences of conservative management of full thickness rotator cuff tears? Will the muscle belly undergo fat atrophy leading to an irreparable tendon?

References

1. Bok K, Sorenson AK, Jorgenson U, Nygaard M, Krarup AL, Thune C, Sloth C, Pederson ST (2010) The value of clinical tests in acute full thickness tear of the supraspinatus tendon: does a subacromial lidocaine injection help in clinical diagnosis? A prospective study. Arthroscopy 26(6):734–742

2. Milano G, Grasso A, Salvatore M, Zarelli D, Deriu L, Fabbriciani C (2007) Arthroscopic rotator cuff repair with and without subacromial decompression: a prospective randomized study. Arthroscopy 23:81–88
3. Gartsmen GM, O'Connor DP (2004) Arthroscopic rotator cuff repair with and without arthroscopic subarcromial decompression: a prospective randomized study of one year outcomes. JBJS 13:424–426
4. Shin SJ, Oh JH, Chung SW, Song MH (2012) The efficacy of acromioplasty in the arthroscopic repair of small- to medium-sized rotator cuff tears without acromial spur: prospective comparative study. Arthroscopy 28(5):628–635
5. Friedman RJ, Bonutti Pm, Genez B (1998) Cine magnetic resonance imaging of the subcoracoid region. Orthopedics 21(5):545–548
6. Tuoheti Y, Itoi E, Pradcaan RL, Wokabayaski I, Takahashi S, Minagawa H, Kobayashi M, Okada K, Shimada Y (2005) Apoptosis in the supraspinatus tendon with stage II subacromial impingement. JSES 14(5):535–541
7. Soifer TB, Leny HJ, Soifer IM, Kleinbart F, Kigorita V, Bryk E (1996) Neurohistology of the subacromial space. Arthroscopy 12(2):182–186

Arthroscopy and Repair

11

Jaap Willems, Dan Guttmann, Guillermo Arce
and Greg Bain

11.1 Partial Cuff Tears

11.1.1 Known Facts

The current literature regarding classification appears to be underpowered for valid conclusions. The comprehensive ISAKOS Rotator Cuff Disease Classification System previously presented at this book will be helpful for research and daily practice guidelines.

At this moment, the weight of evidence supporting a variety of techniques for partial rotator cuff repair is low. Most of the studies are either observational or limited in size.

Outcomes data that firmly support these recommendations are not available; however, these recommendations are of practical importance. Partial tears with greater than 50 % involvement should be repaired, while smaller tears could be managed conservatively with physical therapy and modification of activity. In cases

---

J. Willems (✉)
Hoflaan 22, 1861 CR, Bergen, Netherlands
e-mail: w.j.willems@xs4all.nl; willems.jaap@gmail.com

D. Guttmann
Taos Orthopaedic Institute, 1219-A Gusdorf Road, Taos, NM 87571, USA
e-mail: drg@taosortho.com; drg2812@gmail.com

G. Arce
Department of Orthopaedic Surgery, Instituto Argentino de Diagnóstico y Tratamiento,
Buenos Aires, Argentina
e-mail: guillermorarce@ciudad.com.ar; equipo_arce@yahoo.com

G. Bain
Department of Orthopaedics and Trauma, University of Adelaide, Adelaide, Australia
e-mail: greg@gregbain.com.au

which require surgery, debridement with or without sub-acromial decompression may suffice, rather than a formal repair. Preoperatively, tear depth should be assessed in all partial tears to gain further insight. There are several surgical alternatives for the correction of partial tears, including trans-tendon repair, trans-osseous repair, completion of the tear and either single and/or double row repair.

Internal derangements of the shoulder involving the labrum and/or the biceps tendon do not occur in isolation and should be addressed during the index surgical procedure.

Secondary factors such as SLAP lesions, posterior capsule tightness and/or anterior laxity may play a role in the pathogenesis of partial thickness rotator cuff tears.

Bursal sided partial rotator cuff tears are usually related to acromial spurring and represent a key step in a pathologic cascade that leads to shoulder progressive deterioration.

11.2 Full Thickness Tears

11.2.1 Open Versus Arthroscopic Repairs

In a thorough meta-analysis, arthroscopic rotator cuff repair showed better visualization and allowed for a thorough understanding of the disease and its associated conditions, including biceps and labral pathology; cartilage, capsular and ligamentous alterations. Moreover, arthroscopic repair lead to better identification of arthritis than open surgery. Thus, arthroscopic rotator cuff repair appears to have a significant clinical advantage compared to open repair.

Studies assessing both surgical approaches are limited in size and methodology, providing limited evidence for determining the best treatment option. In addition, improvements in arthroscopic technique occurred after the majority of these studies rendering any conclusion obsolete. Still, arthroscopic repair has the ability to visualize the entire joint-including the rotator cuff-, decreases loss of motion, preserves the deltoid muscle, lowers infection rates and postoperative pain, expedites physical therapy, and shortens hospital stays. Furthermore, long-term functional outcome is better with arthroscopy at the expense of longer operating times, higher total cost for equipment and consumables when compared to open surgery. However, cost is actually offset by reduced cost for analgesics, earlier hospital discharge, rehabilitation and earlier return to work.

Chiefly, arthroscopic superiority over open surgery is observed in small tears, while in large cuff tears, there is no difference between repairing techniques.

11.2.2 Single Versus Double Row Repairs

Comparative data between both techniques (single and double row) is confounded by the use of equivalent numbers of anchors in both techniques. A recently

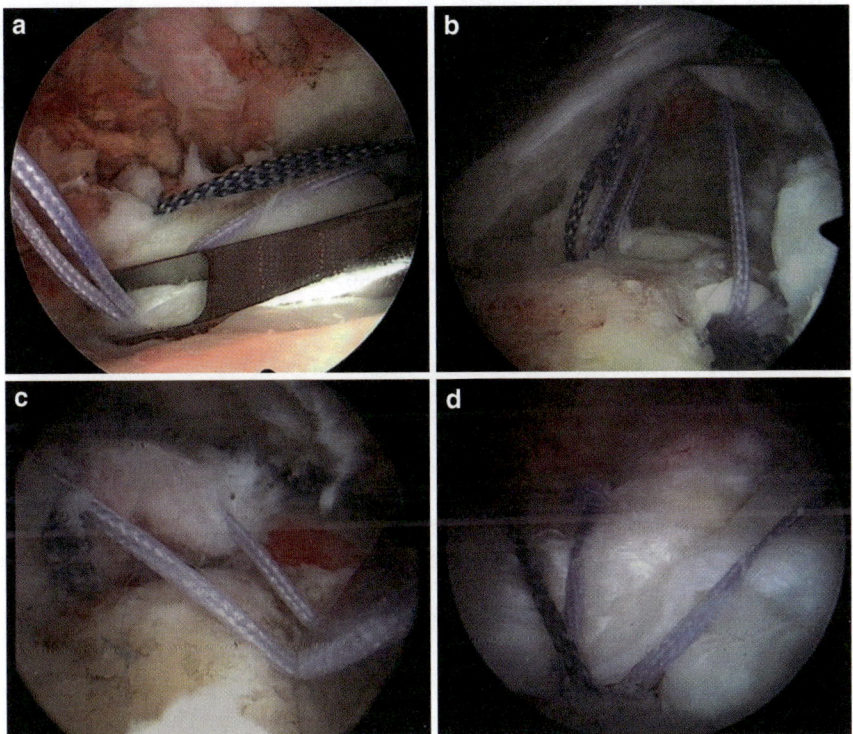

Fig. 11.1 Right Shoulder. Double Row Rotator Cuff Repair viewed arthroscopically. **a** A suture-passing device is introduced. In this step, in order to reduce tension, it is essential to avoid excessive medial sutures through the tendon. **b** Medial row suture anchors (close to the articular cartilage margin) can be seen. **c** The lateral row suture anchor has been delivered without overstretching of the tendon. **d** Final appearance of the procedure illustrating a tensionless reconstruction

reported systematic review suggested that double row repair offers higher initial fixation strength and greater footprint coverage, improves contact pressure, decreases gap formation with higher load to failure than single repair. Nonetheless, these biomechanical advantages did not translate into better clinical outcome. Double row repair appears to be particularly advantageous for large tears (2.5–3.5 cm in size). Recent data suggest that medial recurrent tears can be very difficult to handle, occurring more frequently after double row technique. Thus, surgeons should pay special attention when applying the double row technique to stiff retracted tendons. Over reduction and an increased tension due to the double row fixation technique should be avoid. Figure 11.1. Since double row repairs increases operative time, cost and constitutes a technical challenge to the operator, we recommend its use in carefully selected cases.

11.2.3 Unresolved Issues

Which is the actual healing rate following rotator cuff repair?

Could we predict tear progression and provide a guide for surgical-decision making?

Indications for single versus double row rotator cuff repair.

Does the number of anchors affect negatively tendon healing at the bone site?

Do high tension suture bridge type configuration repairs strangle the tendon, decreasing vascularity and increasing the incidence of type 2 (muscle-tendon junction) failures?

11.3 The Biceps Tendon

11.3.1 Known Facts

The complex biceps-pulley anatomy plays a major role in biceps stability and may be partly responsible for the development of a painful shoulder. Because of its intricate nature, pulley reconstruction is not advised in patients with isolated tear.

Long-term wasting of the long head of the biceps can trigger pain and should be addressed by either tenotomy or tenodesis, depending on the patient's demands and cosmetics. Biceps tenodesis improves cosmetic results and increases elbow flexion and supination strength compared to biceps tenotomy. The biceps is fixed to the proximal humerus with suture anchors or interference screws. Both techniques show successful results without any significant differences between them. Figure 11.2.

Proximal biceps tenodesis is frequently associated with postoperative pain at the groove because it leaves degenerative tendon below the fixation site. Moving distal with the tenodesis may be beneficial to prevent postoperative pain. Preoperatively, palpation of the biceps groove below the pectoralis major (the Mazzocca Sign) may help determine the feasibility and efficacy of subpectoral tenodesis. The latter maneuver is especially relevant given the fact that non-invasive imaging (MRI) cannot establish the most appropriate site for tenodesis.

Visualization of the articular view of the glenohumeral joint and the long head of the biceps tendon by arthroscopy may be insufficient for surgical decisions because the biceps tendon may not be fully appreciated. Thus, it also is important to search for edema on the MRI and attempt to reproduce pain utilizing the Mazzocca Sign and palpating the biceps tendon.

Distal biceps tenodesis could be performed arthroscopically above the pectoralis major tendon (Fig. 11.3) or open at the sub-pectoralis area.

In the event of biceps tendon tears, pulley lesions and/or subluxation, the presence of subscapularis tears should always be entertained.. Moreover, the presence of coracoid impingement should be excluded, and if present, it should be corrected with coracoids decompression along with the subscapsularis repair.

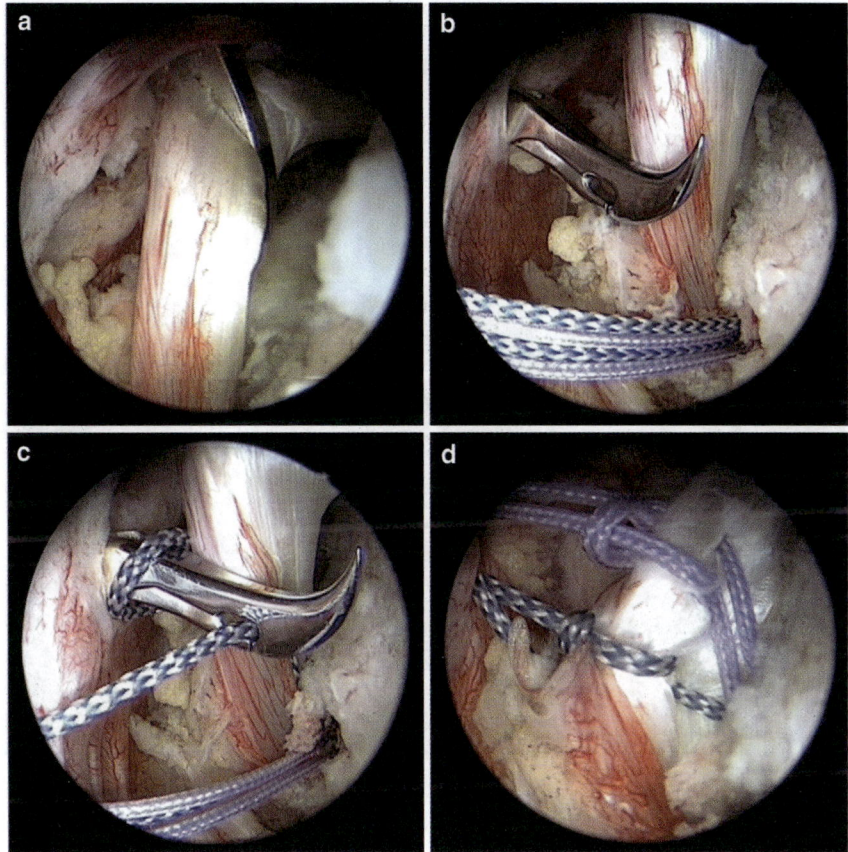

Fig. 11.2 Left Shoulder. Arthroscopic Views of a Biceps Tenodesis performed with suture anchors. **a** Note the long head of the biceps (LHB). **b** A double loaded suture anchor is placed at the bicipital groove. **c** A Lasso Loop Stitch is delivered through the LHB tendon. **d** The LHB is fixed at the proximal humerus

Subscapularis repair may involve a unique rehabilitation, different from the more common repairs of the supraspinatus and infraspinatus.

11.3.2 Unresolved Issues

Timing and location of adjunctive biceps tendon tenodesis during rotator cuff repair (Please see references [1–29] at the end of the chapter).

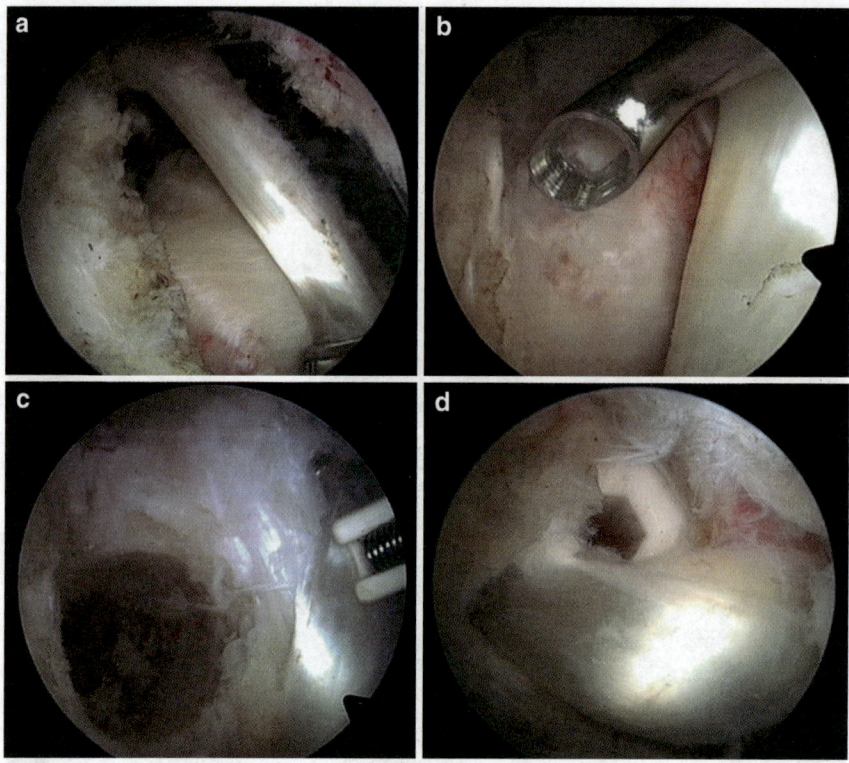

Fig. 11.3 Right Shoulder. Arthroscopic visualization of a distal biceps tenodesis performed with interference screw fixation. **a** The LHB is released from the biceps pulley. **b** A curette is used to debride the bicipital groove removing the sliding zone. **c** An 8-mm wide and 20-mm depth hole is drilled at the lower part of the groove just above the pectoralis major tendon. **d** Final appearance after interference screw fixation

References

1. AAOS (2010) Clinical practice guideline on optimizing the management of rotator cuff problems. American Academy of Orthopaedic Surgeons, Rosemont
2. Baums MH, Buchhorn GH, Spahn G, Poppendieck B, Schultz W, Klinger HM (2008) Biomechanical characteristics of single-row repair in comparison to double-row repair with consideration of the suture configuration and suture material. Knee Surg Sports Traumatol Arthrosc 16:1052–1060
3. Burks RT, Crim J, Brown N, Fink B, Greis PE (2009) A prospective randomized clinical trial comparing arthroscopic single- and double-row rotator cuff repair: magnetic resonance imaging and early clinical evaluation. Am J Sports Med 37:674–682
4. Cho NS, Yi JW, Lee BG, Rhee YG (2010) Retear patterns after arthroscopic rotator cuff repair: single-row versus suture bridge technique. Am J Sports Med 38:664–671
5. Coghlan JA, Buchbinder R, Green S, Johnston RV, Bell SN (2008) Surgery for rotator cuff disease. [Review] [64 refs]. Cochrane Database Syst Rev 1:CD005619

6. Duquin TR, Buyea C, Bisson LJ (2010) Which method of rotator cuff repair leads to the highest rate of structural healing? A systematic review. [Review] [39 refs]. Am J Sports Med 38(4):835–841
7. Franceschi F, Ruzzini L, Longo UG, Martina FM, Zobel BB, Maffulli N et al (2007) Equivalent clinical results of arthroscopic single-row and double-row suture anchor repair for rotator cuff tears: a randomized controlled trial. Am J Sports Med 35:1254–1260
8. Grasso A, Milano G, Salvatore M, Falcone G, Deriu L, Fabbriciani C (2009) Single-row versus double-row arthroscopic rotator cuff repair: a prospective randomized clinical study. Arthroscopy 25:4–12
9. Lorbach O, Bachelier F, Vees J, Kohn D, Pape D (2008) Cyclic loading of rotator cuff reconstructions: single-row repair with modified suture configurations versus double-row repair. Am J Sports Med 36:1504–1510
10. Morse K, Davis AD, Afra R, Kaye EK, Schepsis A, Voloshin I (2008) Arthroscopic versus mini-open rotator cuff repair: a comprehensive review and meta-analysis. [Review] [40 refs]. Am J Sports Med 36(9):1824–1828
11. Nho SJ, Slabaugh MA, Seroyer ST, Grumet RC, Wilson JB, Verma NN et al (2009) Does the literature support double-row suture anchor fixation for arthroscopic rotator cuff repair? A systematic review comparing double-row and single-row suture anchor configuration. [Review] [45 refs]. Arthroscopy 25(11):1319–1328
12. Ozbaydar M, Elhassan B, Esenyel C, Atalar A, Bozdag E, Sunbuloglu E et al (2008) A comparison of single-versus double-row suture anchor techniques in a simulated repair of the rotator cuff: an experimental study in rabbits. J Bone Joint Surg Br 90:1386–1391
13. Prasathaporn N, Kuptniratsaikul S, Kongrukgreatiyos K (2011) Single-row repair versus double-row repair of full-thickness rotator cuff tears. Arthroscopy 27:978–985
14. Saridakis P, Jones G (2010) Outcomes of single-row and double-row arthroscopic rotator cuff repair: a systematic review. [Review] [31 refs]. J Bone Joint Surg Am 92(3):732–742
15. Seida JC, LeBlanc C, Schouten JR, Mousavi SS, Hartling L, Vandermeer B et al (2010) Systematic review: nonoperative and operative treatments for rotator cuff tears. [Review] [81 refs]. Ann Intern Med 153(4):246–255
16. Straus EJ, Salata MJ, Kercher J, Barker JU, McGill K, Bach BR, Romeo AA, Verma NN (2011) The arthroscopic management of partial-thickness rotator cuff tears: a systematic review of the literature. Arthroscopy 27(4):568–580
17. Trantalis JN, Boorman RS, Pletsch K, Lo IK (2008) Medial rotator cuff failure after arthroscopic double-row rotator cuff repair. Arthroscopy 24:727–731
18. Voigt C, Bosse C, Vosshenrich R, Schulz AP, Lill H (2010) Arthroscopic supraspinatus tendon repair with suture-bridging technique: functional outcome and magnetic resonance imaging. Am J Sports Med 38:983–991
19. Yamakado K, Katsuo S, Mizuno K, Arakawa H, Hayashi S (2010) Medial-row failure after arthroscopic double-row rotator cuff repair. Arthroscopy 26:430–435
20. Ball C, Galatz LM, Yamaguchi K (2001) Tenodesis or tenotomy of the biceps tendon: why and when to do it. Tech Shoulder Elbow Surg 2:140–152
21. Boileau P, Neyton L (2005) Arthroscopic tenodesis for the long head of the biceps. Oper Orthop Traumatol 17(6):601–623
22. Hsu A, Ghodadra N, Provencher M, Lewis P, Bach B (2011) Biceps tenotomy versus tenodesis: a review of clinical outcomes and biomechanical results. J Shoulder Elbow Surg 20:326–332
23. Mariani PP, Bellelli A, Botticella C (1997) Arthroscopic absence of the long head of the biceps tendon. Arthroscopy 13:499–501
24. Mazzocca AD, Bicos J, Santangelo S, Romeo AA, Arciero RA (2005) The biomechanical evaluation of four fixation techniques for proximal biceps tenodesis. Arthroscopy 21(11):1296–1306
25. Sanders B, Lavery K, Pennington S, Warner JJP (2008) Biceps tendon tenodesis: success with proximal versus distal fixation. Arthroscopy 24(6):e9

26. Slenker N, Lawson K, Cicciotti M, Dodson C, Cohen S (2012) Biceps tenotomy versus tenodesis. Clinical outcomes. Arthroscopy 28(4):576–582
27. Walch G, Nové-Josserand L, Boileau P, Levigne C (1998) Subluxations and dislocations of the tendon of the long head biceps. J Shoulder Elbow Surg 7:100–108
28. Wolf RS, Zheng N, Weichel D (2005) Long head biceps tenotomy versus tenodesis: a cadaveric biomechanical analysis. Arthroscopy 21:182–185
29. Bennet W (2004) Arthroscopic bicipital sheath repair: two-year follow-up with pulley lesions. Arthroscopy 20:964–973

Augments and Prosthesis

12

Felix Savoie III, John Uribe, Matthew Provencher, Francisco Vergara and Emilio Calvo

12.1 Known Facts

The best results come from anatomic restoration of the normal shoulder anatomy. Most tears are amenable to repair with modern techniques. Biologic and mechanical enhancement of rotator cuff repair surgery remains a viable goal of all surgeons. Current advances in laboratory technology have shown to promote tendon healing but its precise role during rotator cuff repair is currently under investigation.

F. Savoie III (✉)
Tulane University School of Medicine, 1430 Tulane Avenue, SL32,
New Orleans, LA 70112, USA
e-mail: fsavoie@tulane.edu

J. Uribe
UHZ Sports Medicine Institute, 1150 Campo Sano Avenue, Suite 200,
Coral Gables, FL 33146, USA
e-mail: johnu@baptisthealth.net

M. Provencher
Naval Medical Center San Diego, 455 B Ave, Coronado, CA 92118, USA
e-mail: mattprovencher@earthlink.net

F. Vergara
MEDS Sport Medicine Center, Isabel La Catolica 3740 Las Condes,
Parque 12650 casa 24 Lo Barnechea, 755-0557, Santiago, Chile
e-mail: franciscoverg@gmail.com

E. Calvo
Shoulder and Elbow Reconstructive Surgery Unit, Department of Orthopedic Surgery,
Fundacion Jimenez Diaz—Capio, Av. Reyes Catolicos 2, 28040, Madrid, Spain
e-mail: ecalvo@fjd.es; emilio.calvo@gmail.com

The use of platelet-rich plasma or autologous pluri-potential biologic cells in rotator cuff healing constitutes two promising strategies for healing purposes. At this moment, there is substantial heterogeneity in harvest systems in terms of the amount of material that is delivered to the tendon. In addition, there are technical limitations to avoid washout of treatment cells at the repair site. Experimental studies have shown that different growth factors are capable of increasing the strength of repairs. Unfortunately, this seems to be accomplished through an increase in scar tissue production instead of by forming a physiological tendon-to-bone insertion. The optimal timing, concentration, and combination of the different growth factors is still unclear. As in transduced and modified stem cell applications, the optimal dosage and vehicle for delivery has remained elusive.

To deliver leukocyte and platelet concentrates seems to be a promising approach to biological augmentation of rotator cuff tears, as these concentrates contain many of the fundamental growth factors at high dosages, can release the growth factors over time, and can be a potential carrier for stem cell application. Matrix metalloproteinase-3 (MMP-3) is an enzyme involved in the breakdown of extracellular matrix in normal physiological processes and plays a major role in tendon tissue degeneration and remodelling. The use of gene therapy to target MMP-3 and enhance tendon healing is a tantalizing area of current and future research. In spite of these promising findings, randomized comparative clinical studies have failed to demonstrate any beneficial effect of all these biologic therapeutic interventions. Further research is needed to define the correct dosage, quantification, and timing, and to fully understand the teamwork between modified stem cells and different growth factors.

To promote tendon healing some investigators have used mechanical patches or scaffolds with varying results. The rationale for using these devices may include mechanical augmentation or biologically enhancing tendon healing. The ideal scaffold material would serve as an inductive template, with optimal mechanical properties to prevent or limit tendon retear during the process of degradation, engraftment, and remodelling, resulting in an integration and reconstruction of the tissue. Unfortunately, the devices currently available may not provide all of these capabilities. The use of non-cross linked autograft tissue seems to provide the best solution. The clinical use of any scaffold for bridging or interposition is still a matter of debate. Since most of rotator cuff tears can be repaired with proper surgical technique, the use of these devices are usually recommended for massive retracted irreparable tears that cannot be reconstructed with low tension, but they could also be employed as augmentation devices in smaller tears with poor tissue quality. Although synthetic patches hold promise, there are little clinical data to demonstrate the appropriate indications, efficacy and adverse effects of scaffolds for rotator cuff repairs. Combination strategies, like tissue-engineered constructs that mate scaffolds with growth factors or pluripotential biologic cells may meet the goals of these therapies.

The use of tendon transfer in massive tears with concomitant atrophy seems a reasonable strategy for supplementation but limited to selected cases. Tendon transfers are mainly indicated in relatively young patients with irreparable rotator cuff tears in whom reverse prosthesis is contraindicated. Latissimus dorsi transfer could represent a feasible strategy in a patient with an intact subscapsularis, acceptable passive flexion, and a large posterior superior tear and severe atrophy. Moreover, partial or complete subcoracoid pectoralis major transfer may be an attractive solution in a patient with an intact infraspinatus and a severely torn, atrophic and non reparable subscapularis. Adherence to postoperative rehabilitation remains crucial to the success of these procedures, as well as to deltoid integrity and tendon quality. The management of combined anterior and postero-superior defects continues to be a difficult problem. Although some reports have suggested the benefits of combined pectoralis with latissimus dorsi tendon transfer, data are very scant.

The main indication for reverse shoulder arthroplasty in patients with rotator cuff tears is the presence of rotator cuff-tear arthropathy. Reverse shoulder arthroplasty has proven to be very successful in this condition, with substantial improvements in pain and active elevation. Recently, the indications for reverse shoulder arthroplasty have been expanded to include selected massive cuff tears with pseudoparalysis but no arthritis with good results. In this situation, the use of reverse shoulder prosthesis during rotator cuff repair should be limited to elderly patients with painful shoulders, truly irreparable tear, severe muscular atrophy, pseudoparalysis and anterior superior escape with a positive lag sign.

The use of reverse shoulder prosthesis during rotator cuff repair should be limited to elderly patients with painful shoulders, truly irreparable tear (Goutallier stage 4), pseudoparalysis and anterior superior escape with a positive lag sign. In order to restore external rotation in individuals with a positive lag sign adjunctive Latissimus Dorsi (LD) with or without Teres Major (TM) transfer is probably advisable. When using the Gerber technique, transferring the LD to the greater tuberosity in RSA, only the LD is commonly used. When performing the Episcopo technique, just redirecting the tendon around the humerus, it is technically difficult to use only the LD and generally both TM as well as LD are used.

12.2 Areas of Future Research

Determination of the best method to acquire and process autologous pluripotential cells to enhance healing.

Determine the best method for local delivery and maintenance of pluripotential cells within the healing zone of the rotator cuff.

Determine the best method to inhibit tendon tissue degradation

Evaluate the potential clinical benefits of biologic therapeutic interventions in rotator cuff tear repairs.

In-vitro and animal studies are warranted to determine the proper role of augmentation devices during rotator cuff surgery.

Analyze the long-term outcome of reverse shoulder arthroplasty in patients with massive irreparable rotator cuff tears without osteoarthritis (Please see references [1–10] at the end of the chapter).

References

1. Butler DL, Juncosa-Melvin N, Boivin GP, Galloway MT, Shearn JT, Gooch C et al (2008) Functional tissue engineering for tendon repair: A multidisciplinary strategy using mesenchymal stem cells, bioscaffolds, and mechanical stimulation. J Orthop Res 26:1–9
2. Lopez-Vidriero E, Goulding KA, Simon DA, Sanchez M, Johnson DH (2010) The use of platelet-rich plasma in arthroscopy and sports medicine: optimizing the healing environment. Arthroscopy 26:269–278
3. Bergeson AG, Tashjian RZ, Greis PE, Crim J, Stoddard GJ, Burks RT (2012) Effects of platelet-rich fibrin matrix on repair integrity of at-risk rotator cuff tears. Am J Sports Med 40:286–293
4. Shea KP, McCarthy MB, Ledgard F, Arciero C, Chowaniec D, Mazzocca AD (2010) Human tendon cell response to 7 commercially available extracellular matrix materials: an in vitro study. Arthroscopy 26:1181–1188
5. Derwin KA, Baker AR, Spragg RK, Leigh DR, Ianotti JP (2006) Commercial extracellular matrix scaffolds for rotator cuff tendon repair: Biomechanical, biochemical, and cellular properties. J Bone Joint Surg Am 88: 2665–2672
6. Gerber C, Maquieira G, Espinosa N (2006) Latissimus dorsi transfer for the treatment of irreparable rotator cuff tears. J Bone Joint Surg Am 88:113–120
7. Resch H, Povacz P, Ritter E, Matschi W (2000) Transfer of the pectoralis major muscle for the treatment of irreparable rupture of the subscapularis tendon. J Bone Joint Surg Am 82:372–382
8. Guery J, Favard L, Sirveaux F, Oudet D, Mole D, Walch G (2006) Reverse total shoulder arthroplasty. Survivorship analysis of eighty replacements followed for five to ten years. J Bone Joint Surg Am 88:1742–1747
9. Mulieri P, Dunning P, Klein S, Pupello D, Frankle M (2010) Reverse shoulder arthroplasty for the treatment of irreparable rotator cuff tear without glenohumeral artritis. J Bone Joint Surg Am 92:2544–2556
10. Boileau P, Chuinard C, Roussanne Y, Bicknell RT, Rochet N, Trojani C (2008) Reverse shoulder arthroplasty combined with a modified latissimus dorsi and teres major tendon transfer for shoulder pseudoparalysis associated with dropping qrm. Clin Orthop Relat Res 466:584–593